S0-ACG-384

MED. SCHOOL

Norris and Campbell's

Anaesthetics, Resuscitation and Intensive Care

Norris and Campbell's Anaesthetics, Resuscitation and Intensive Care

Donald Campbell
MB, ChB, FFARCS, DA
Professor of Anaesthesia, University of Glasgow
Honorary Consultant Anaesthetist, Glasgow Royal
Infirmary

Alastair A. Spence
MD, FFARCS
Reader in Anaesthesia, University of Glasgow
Honorary Consultant Anaesthetist, Western
Infirmary, Glasgow

Foreword by

John W. Dundee
MD, PhD, FFARCS, FFARCSI
Professor of Anaesthetics, the Queen's University,
Belfast

FIFTH EDITION

CHURCHILL LIVINGSTONE
EDINBURGH LONDON AND NEW YORK 1978

CHURCHILL LIVINGSTONE
Medical Division of Longman Group Limited

Distributed in the United States of America by
Churchill Livingstone Inc., 19 West 44th Street, New York,
N.Y. 10036 and by associated companies, branches
and representatives throughout the world.

© Longman Group Limited 1978

All rights reserved. No part of this publication may
be reproduced, stored in a retrieval system, or
transmitted in any form or by any means, electronic,
mechanical, photocopying, recording or otherwise,
without the prior permission of the publishers
(Churchill Livingstone, Robert Stevenson House,
1–3 Baxter's Place, Leith Walk, Edinburgh, EH1 3AF).

First Edition   1965
Second Edition   1968
Third Edition   1971
    Reprinted   1972
Fourth Edition   1974
Fifth Edition   1978
    Reprinted   1979

ISBN 0 443 01573 2

British Library Cataloguing in Publication Data
Norris, Walter
    Norris and Campbell's anaesthetics,
    resuscitation and intensive care.—5th ed.
    1. Anesthesia
    I. Campbell, Donald, b. 1930   II. Spence,
    Alastair A   III. Anaesthetics, resuscitation
    and intensive care
    617' .96   RD81   78–40130

Printed in Hong Kong by Wah Cheong Printing Press Ltd

Foreword

In recommending a book for use by medical students and housemen one should perhaps justify their learning something about anaesthesia and its ever widening field of non-theatre activities.

In many parts of the English-speaking world, general anaesthesia is now in the hands of specialist or trainee-specialist anaesthetists. While the advantages of this cannot be overemphasised from both the surgeon's and patient's point of view, it is unfortunate that, in Great Britain at least, the newly qualified doctor gets little opportunity of handling and caring for the anaesthetised patient. Most undergraduates simply fulfil the requirements of their particular medical school with regard to the administration of anaesthetics and are naturally unwilling to devote more than the minimum time to the subject in an already overcrowded curriculum. Thus they miss an opportunity of gaining first-hand experience of dealing with patients who have been made comatose and who may have induced respiratory or circulatory depression. There is no place where these states, which require the urgent attention of every doctor, can be seen so frequently and where their treatment is so successful as during anaesthesia or the immediate post-operative period.

No book can fill the place of practical experience in the operating room, recovery ward, intensive care, and respiratory units, but Drs Norris and Campbell have prepared the present volume so that the limited time which can be allocated to anaesthesia and allied topics will be spent to the best advantage. It contains a clear concise account of the different types of anaesthesia and the simplest and most reliable means by which these can be produced. Such a text could so easily develop into a 'do it yourself' recipe book, but the authors have avoided this temptation by including adequate data on the pertinent physiology and pharmacology.

On such a sound foundation, the writers have based a valuable section on modern methods of resuscitation. This alone could recommend the book not only to students and house staff but to all physicians who are becoming increasingly aware of the immediate treatment of cardiovascular collapse. While avoiding controversial topics, this section deals fully with such important aspects as pH control and is presented with such clarity and simplicity as to be helpful to readers of all types.

The anaesthetist should be in a particularly favourable position with regard to knowledge on relief of post-operative pain. Drs Norris and Campbell have included precise instructions on the management of this important topic which will save many embarrassing moments for the 'houseman' and be of inestimable value to the patient. Although it would take a book many times the size of the present one to deal adequately with all aspects of analgesia and pain relief, the basic knowledge in the present volume is a good foundation on which interested doctors could build such information. As the anaesthetist's interest in the patient should start with his pre-operative preparation and ordering of pre-anaesthetic medication, so this book covers all topics from the drugs given before operation to the long-term management of respiratory insufficiency.

It is not surprising that since the majority of anaesthetic textbooks cater for the potential specialist they contain too much detail for other readers. In addition they usually present both sides of controversial arguments, necessitating some experience in understanding the various views expressed and their relevance to the circumstances under which the reader may be working. This defect is avoided in the present volume which is a valuable book not only for senior medical students and house surgeons or house physicians but a useful manual for the beginner in the first few months of his anaesthetic training.

Belfast, 1965   JOHN W. DUNDEE

Professor Campbell is fortunate in having secured help from Dr A. A. Spence in preparing the latest edition of this book following the untimely death of Dr Walter Norris. This volume has now been firmly established as a most useful book, not only for medical students, but also for beginners in Anaesthesia and for paramedicals involved in intensive care.

Belfast, 1978   J. W. D.

Preface to the Fifth Edition

The untimely death of my friend and co-author, Dr Walter Norris, occurred shortly after the publication of the fourth edition of this book. The continuation of this work, to which he devoted so much time and energy over the years, has been assured however since Dr Alastair A. Spence has consented to join me in the production of this present edition and and future editions. We hope that, while an extensive revision of the material has been undertaken on this occasion, the original aim has not been lost sight of and this book will continue to provide a useful introductory text for students, residents and specialist nursing staff.

Glasgow, 1978　　　　　　　　　　　　　　　　　D. CAMPBELL

Preface to the First Edition

The administration of anaesthetics in this country is now firmly established in the hands of the specialist anaesthetist. Indeed after qualification a doctor may never require to give an anaesthetic again if he does not wish to do so. Most doctors, however, in their hospital life and indeed outwith hospital, will at some time work in co-operation with members of the anaesthetic department staff. Surgeons, obstetricians and dentists, of course, are in daily contact with anaesthetists, physicians are meeting and working with them in the treatment of various chest diseases, and many other specialists also co-operate with them.

To the student we hope to offer a background to his practical teaching in the operating theatre and explain the 'whys' of anaesthesia rather than to attempt to explain how to give an anaesthetic. If he wishes to learn how to give an anaesthetic, he must do this in the operating theatre and over the course of many weeks or even months. We hope also to show that the interests and work of the anaesthetist are not limited to the operating theatre.

To the resident in hospital we hope to explain how he may help the anaesthetist and thus his patients by careful pre-operative care of the patient and by thinking of the therapy he is using and the effect it may have on the anaesthetic later. We hope also he will realise that there are many ways in which the anaesthetist can help him and that there are times when he should call a consultant anaesthetist rather than a consultant surgeon or physician.

In many hospitals the resident will find himself dealing with patients in intensive care units, particularly those dealing with respiratory emergencies, both medical and surgical. This is a field of work where it is essential that everyone should know what is expected of him and what can be done to help severely disabled patients. It is essential that 'the man on the spot' should be fully conversant with all the methods which are used.

No matter what path the student intends to follow, we feel that a thorough knowledge of methods of resuscitation will prove invaluable to him whether he practises in hospital, in general practice or in any other branch of medicine. Acute respiratory and cardiac failure may occur anywhere and the chance of survival of the patient depends entirely on the ability of those present to maintain or restart an efficient circulation and ventilation within a few minutes.

It is for this reason that we have dealt with resuscitation, intensive care, tracheal intubation and intravenous therapy in greater practical detail. As with the administration of anaesthetics, however, there is no substitute for practical training and experience.

Finally, we feel that a knowledge of the accidents and medico-legal hazards which are associated with anaesthesia, resuscitation and intensive care will impress on both students and residents the need for care in applying these techniques.

Glasgow, 1965   W. NORRIS
                                                 D. CAMPBELL

Acknowledgements

We are grateful to Professor John W. Dundee who has so kindly written the foreword to this book.

Dr A. R. Aitkenhead, Dr Kirsteen Dewar and Dr A. G. Macdonald provided valuable help in the preparation of the manuscript.

To Professor Alex. C. Forrester we are indebted for the chapter he has contributed and for his encouragement.

For permission to reproduce illustrations, we are grateful to:

Messrs E. & S. Livingstone: Figs 3.14, 3.15, 7.1, 9.9, 16.1, 16.2, 16.3, 16.4, 16.5 and some forty illustrations from *A Nurse's Guide to Anaesthetics, Resuscitation and Intensive Care* (6th edition 1976)

Macmillan Journals Ltd, publishers of the *British Journal of Anaesthesia* and Drs G. M. Paterson, G. H. Hulands and Professor John Nunn: Fig. 3.6

The Editor of *The British Medical Bulletin* and Dr H. G. Epstein: Fig. 3.7

The Editor of the *Proceedings of the Royal Society of Medicine* and Professor W. A. Mackey: Figs 12.5, 12.6 and 12.7

We also acknowledge gratefully the following who supplied us with illustrations or material for their production:

The British Oxygen Company Limited: Figs 3.2, 3.3, 3.13, 5.3, 8.3, 8.4, 8.8, 8.9, 13.1 and 15.1

Brunswick Corporation (U.K.) Ltd: Fig. 6.2

Smith and Nephew—Southalls Ltd: Fig. 6.3

Professor Alex. C. Forrester: Figs 6.11 and 10.5 and the illustrations in his chapter

Portland Plastics Ltd: Figs 8.7 and 11.3

Messrs Medical and Industrial Equipment Ltd: Figs 8.15 and 13.2

Mr Gabriel Donald and Dr A. B. M. Telfer: Fig. 18.3

Department of Medical Illustrations, Western Infirmary, Glasgow: Figs 1.5, 3.16, 5.1, 6.8 and 6.9

Macmillan Journals Ltd and the Editor of *Nursing Times*: Fig. 5.2

Abbot Laboratories: Fig. 13.3

Dr Nimmo McKellar: Fig. 18.1

Macarthys Ltd: Fig. 19.5

Dr G. Teasdale and the Editor of the *Journal of the Royal College of Physicians*: Fig. 11.13

Dr E. I. Eger and the Editor of *Anesthesiology*: Fig. 1.6

The Editor of *Anaesthesia* and Dr J. G. Bourne: Fig. 1.4

The Warning Notice before the Appendix is reproduced by permission of the Scottish Home and Health Department.

We are again indebted to Mr Robin Callander for the time, patience and skill he has devoted to producing the diagrams and line drawings. The photographs are the work of the late Mr Kelly, Mr Burns and the staff of the Department of Medical Illustration, Glasgow Royal Infirmary, to whom we are also indebted for their time, patience and skill.

Finally, we acknowledge our gratitude to our secretaries Miss E. Polley, Mrs M. MacLeod and Mrs R. Ottaway.

Contents

1

Basic concepts

Analgesia means absence of pain and is a term used to describe the state in which pain has been abolished but other sensations remain, and the patient is conscious.

Anaesthesia means absence of all sensation; the term implies that the patient is unconscious and all sensation is lost.

The conduction of painful impulses to the brain from a site of injury may be interrupted at one of several points between the origin and the sensory cortex (Fig. 1.1). We are concerned with the use of drugs which do this, but these impulses may be interrupted also by cutting the nerves or by the surgical division of a tract in the spinal cord. Such surgical intervention may be helpful in alleviating the pain of incurable malignant disease. Tumours

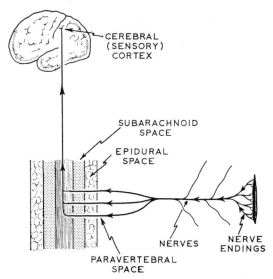

Fig. 1.1 The Pathway of Pain: the course of painful impulses from a wound to the brain is illustrated. The passage of the impulse can be interrupted at any of the sites indicated by the arrows.

themselves may interrupt the passage of impulses, by producing ischaemia, as will injury to a nerve, for example following a fracture. Extreme cold can block nerve conduction also.

Many drugs relieve pain without having any specific effect on the nervous system; for example salicylates ease pain because they reduce inflammation; cytotoxic drugs may reduce pain by causing regression of a tumour.

The drugs which relieve pain by an action on the nervous system may be classified as follows:

Drugs acting on the central nervous system. These act by depressing the brain which receives the impulses so that the pain is felt either with diminished intensity or not at all. Of course these drugs are not brought into contact with the brain by direct injection, but are carried to the brain by the blood stream. They may be administered via the stomach, the bowel, the lungs, or they may be injected into a vein directly.

Drugs acting on the peripheral nervous system (local analgesics). These drugs block conduction in nerve fibres and are deposited close to the nerves which are to be blocked. A local anaesthetic may be injected directly in close proximity to the nerve, or it may be injected at some distance from the nerve, being carried to the fibre either under the influence of gravity or by diffusion in the cerebrospinal fluid following subarachnoid injection. In all of these situations, however, there is a local or regional effect only.

GENERAL ANAESTHESIA

Anaesthesia involves the abolition of all sensation, of touch, posture, temperature and pain, and is the term normally reserved for states in which the patient is unconscious. Many of the modern techniques of anaesthesia are complex in respect of both the range of drugs and the equipment used. However, it is best to begin by considering the simple and traditional method of producing anaesthesia with a single drug. A large number of drugs are capable of abolishing all sensation, but some such as methyl alcohol can be expected to produce permanent tissue damage, while others such as ethyl alcohol, although less damaging to tissues, are associated with a prolonged and unpleasant recovery. The relatively small group of drugs known as the *inhalation anaesthetics,* for example diethylether ('ether'), chloroform, or halothane, produce reversible depression of the central nervous system with a quality of recovery that is acceptable to the patient.

Figure 1.2 shows examples of simple anaesthetic techniques for a mouse and a man respectively. In both cases, the primary objective is to achieve a sufficient concentration of the anaesthetic in the central nervous system so that, by depressing it, the mouse or the man will not move in response to a stimulus such as incision of the skin.

In both examples, the inspired gas of the subject (the gaseous environment) must contain not only molecules of the anaesthetic agent, but also a concentration of oxygen sufficient to maintain life. Moreover, the expired carbon dioxide must not contribute significantly to the next breath. Thus, the inspired gas must be as 'fresh' as possible for each breath.

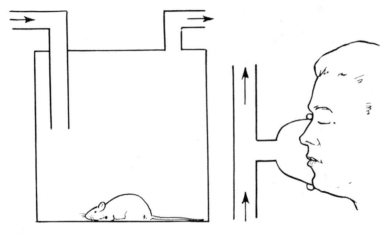

Fig. 1.2

The transfer of anaesthetic molecules to the brain occurs via the lungs and the pulmonary and arterial circulation. Of course, the anaesthetic is distributed to all the tissues of the body in addition to the central nervous system. Although this is inevitable, in many instances it is undesirable since many anaesthetics have known adverse side effects, such as myocardial depression. The transfer of molecules from one phase to another (gaseous environment to lung, lung to blood, etc.) can occur only if there is a partial pressure or tension gradient from one phase to another (Fig. 1.3). In a gas mixture, the partial pressure of one of the components is the product of the percentage concentration and the total ambient pressure. Thus, at normal atmospheric pressure

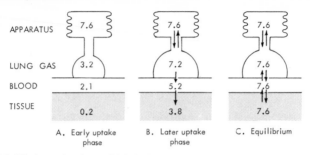

Fig. 1.3 (A) An early phase of inhalation anaesthetic in which the lung gas partial pressure of the anaesthetic (halothane in this case) is less than that of the delivery system (apparatus) but greater than that of the blood or tissue. Net transfer is in one direction. (B) The lung gas is almost equilibriated with the system but blood and tissue lag behind. Net transfer continues. (C) Equilibriation across all compartments. No net transfer.

(760 mmHg or 101.3 kPa), the partial pressure of 1 per cent of halothane will be 1 kPa approximately. The partial pressure or tension of gases in liquid such as blood or other tissues may be defined as the partial pressure which that gas would exert in a gas mixture which is in equilibrium with the liquid. When the transfer of gas molecules across the various phases of the body is complete, there is partial pressure equilibrium. Thereafter, although molecules continue to move at random from one phase to another, there is no *net* exchange from one phase to another.

Uptake and elimination patterns

Figure 1.4 shows the pattern of uptake to equilibrium by the lung alveoli and brain following the administration of six inhalation anaesthetics and nitrogen. Note the different rates at which the partial pressure in the brain approaches equilibrium with the partial pressure in the inspired gas. Although there are many reasons for the differences between these uptake curves, the dominant factor is the difference in lipid solubility, nitrous oxide being poorly soluble and diethylether being highly soluble. A similar set of curves can be produced for the elimination of these agents when the inspired partial pressure has been restored to zero (the anaesthetic has been discontinued), the poorly soluble agents being eliminated rapidly.

Figure 1.5 shows a family of curves (theoretical) for the uptake of halothane to equilibrium at three different inspired partial pressures. The interrupted line shows the uptake pattern which might be employed during the administration of an anaesthetic; the inspired partial pressure may be set to a higher level than that with which the brain would be required to equilibrate, so that the

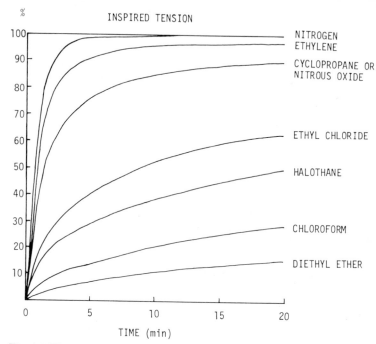

Fig. 1.4 Time course of changes in the lung alveolar concentration of seven anaesthetic gases and nitrogen related to the inspired concentration (100%).

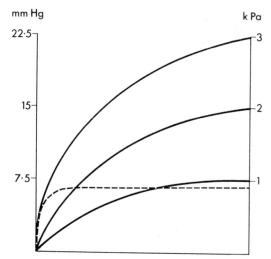

Fig. 1.5 Family of curves (———) showing progress towards equilibrium of a body tissue (brain for example) for three different inspired tensions of halothane (vertical axis mmHg or kPa). The interrupted line shows what is likely to occur during a typical anaesthetic when the vaporizer setting is set first to a high value and reduced gradually.

brain concentration would reach the required level faster than would be possible if the inspired concentration were maintained at a constant level throughout. This device of giving a large 'loading' dose is familiar in many types of drug administration, for example 'digitilisation'. The accepted term for this in anaesthetic practice is *overpressure*.

'Potency and dosage'—the concept of MAC

Doctors are accustomed to thinking of the administration of drugs in terms of a recommended dose range and it may be asked how the *dose* of an inhalation anaesthetic can be determined. Consider a situation in which the tissues of a healthy patient are in equilibrium with a known partial pressure or tension of halothane which just causes sufficient depression of the brain that the patient does not move in response to incision of the skin. The concentration of halothane in the brain tissue, determined by the tension and the solubility in the brain of halothane, may be calculated and expressed as mmol/100 g brain. It is perhaps reassuring to know that the anaesthetist does not undertake such calculations routinely! However, the important point is that approximately the same concentration of halothane in the brain of almost any patient in a similar state of health will produce the same depth of anaesthesia. Indeed, as a general rule, the same concentration would probably produce about the same depth of anaesthesia in many other species, for example the mouse which we considered earlier.

It can be shown that for halothane, the inspired concentration which we have been considering is 0.8 per cent at sea level, or 6 mmHg (0.8 kPa) at any altitude. This is called the *Minimum Alveolar Concentration* (*MAC*) for halothane.

All the inhalation anaesthetic agents have MAC values, the significance of which is the same as in the example of halothane; some of these are given in Table 1.1. There is an approximately inverse linear relationship between MAC for an inhalation anaesthetic, and its lipid solubility (Fig. 1.6).

Those who are mathematically minded will have realised that the depth of anaesthesia would appear to depend on the molecular concentration of the anaesthetic in the brain, rather than any individual property of one drug as compared with another. Thus, MAC is the best description of the dose value for an inhalation anaesthetic. It must be remembered, however, that MAC presumes equilibrium between brain and inspired gas. Already, we have outlined the events preceding the state of equilibrium. Among other factors, we have seen that the time necessary to

Table 1.1. Some properties of the inhalation anaesthetics

	Boiling point (°C)	MAC (% of 1 atm)	Blood/gas partition coefficient
Chloroform	61	—	10.3
Cyclopropane	−34	9.2	0.46
Diethylether	35	1.92	15
Enflurane	56.5	1.68	1.9
Halothane	50	0.75	2.3
Methoxyflurane	104.8	0.16	13.0
Nitrous oxide	−89	105	0.47

achieve equilibrium varies greatly between agents, being only a few minutes for nitrous oxide and more than 30 minutes for diethylether. Such considerations may be very important in determining the suitability of a drug in a specific clinical situation.

We are now in a position to consider what is meant by the *potency* of an inhalation anaesthetic. Textbooks of pharmacology are often rather confusing in this matter, implying that some molecules have a more potent effect on the brain than have others. We have explained why this is unlikely to be so.

A drug such as nitrous oxide (MAC 800 mmHg, 106.6 kPa) which has a low lipid solubility, must be given in high concentrations to achieve any obvious clinical effect. Indeed, surgical anaesthesia cannot be produced with nitrous oxide even at the maximum partial pressure which can be obtained at normal atmospheric pressure. Thus, there are limitations to the use of nitrous oxide as an anaesthetic and it may be described loosely as having a low potency as compared with halothane (MAC = 0.8 kPa). However, the discerning reader will realise that this is a reflection of solubility in tissues rather than an intrinsic pharmacological action of the molecules.

Fractions of MAC may be combined. Thus, as an approximation, one half of the MAC value of nitrous oxide, 53.3 kPa (approximately 50 per cent at sea level), combined with one half MAC of halothane, 0.4 kPa (0.4 per cent), will provide surgical anaesthesia when equilibrium between inspired gas and brain has been achieved.

The components of anaesthesia
Anaesthesia has three components, hypnosis, analgesia and muscular relaxation. In the past, it was common practice to produce all three by the administration of potent inhalation agents such as diethylether, cyclopropane or chloroform, and it is possible to

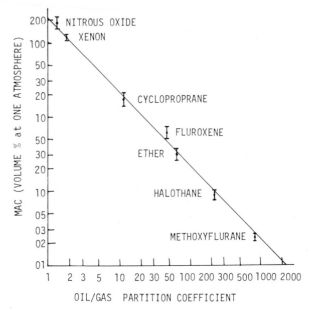

Fig. 1.6 Relationship between oil/gas partition coefficient (an index of lipid solubility) and MAC for seven anaesthetic agents.

do this with halothane, methoxyflurane and enflurane also. However, with the introduction by Griffith and Johnson of Montreal, in 1942, of tubocurarine (curare) to anaesthetic practice, Gray in Liverpool suggested the *triad* of anaesthesia as listed above. Since the unconscious patient does not 'feel' pain in the normally accepted sense, but shows reflex responses to it, 'analgesia' is often replaced by 'suppression of reflex activity' in the triad. It is in this context that the term analgesia is used in this book when we are considering the unconscious patient. By using small doses of specific drugs to produce separately hypnosis , analgesia and muscular relaxation, it is possible to provide the appropriate combination for each patient.

Hypnosis

It is usual to induce hypnosis by intravenous injection of a drug which has a short duration of action; thiopentone and Althesin are the most popular agents but there are several others. Alternatively, one may induce unconsciousness with a gas such as nitrous oxide or cyclopropane or vapours of agents such as halothane or ether. During anaesthesia, hypnosis is maintained by the inhalation of nitrous oxide mixed with oxygen with, where necessary, the addition of a more potent volatile agent such as halothane.

Analgesia

A significant degree of analgesia may be obtained by the inhalation of nitrous oxide in oxygen but this may be supplemented by the addition of volatile agents such as trichlorethylene, ether, halothane or methoxyflurane or by the intravenous injection of an analgesic such as morphine. Where a patient is allowed to breathe spontaneously, a volatile agent is usually employed to supplement nitrous oxide and oxygen. When ventilation is controlled and muscular relaxation obtained by using a drug which blocks the myoneural junction specifically, some anaesthetists prefer to supplement nitrous oxide and oxygen with intravenous agents.

Muscular relaxation

Some degree of muscular relaxation is necessary for most operations. This may vary from simple relaxation of the forearm muscles, during manipulation of a Colles' fracture, to more profound muscular paralysis for upper abdominal and intrathoracic operations. Although muscular relaxation could be produced by the use of one of the more potent volatile anaesthetic agents, the quantities which would be needed would cause a delayed recovery and risk toxicity. Therefore, one of a range of myoneural blocking drugs is employed. These act by antagonising the effect of acetylcholine at the muscle end-plate. A consequence of their use is failure of the muscles of respiration. Thus artificial ventilation has to be instituted, by intermittent positive pressure via a tracheal tube.

The introduction of tubocurarine to anaesthetic practice brought the need for a wide range of skills in respiratory care and detailed understanding of pulmonary and cardiovascular physiology. It is probably true to say that the growth of anaesthesia as a specialty, and the later involvement of the anaesthetist in respiratory intensive care units, stemmed primarily from this development.

Mode of action of anaesthetics

No-one knows precisely how the drugs which produce general anaesthesia act or whether they all act at the same site or sites within the central nervous system, although there are many theories. Elucidation of this complex problem remains as one of the great challenges to medical science and is the subject of active research programmes by many anaesthetists and pharmacologists throughout the world.

LOCAL OR REGIONAL ANALGESIA

Local analgesic drugs

It is known that the passage of impulses along nerves is associated with electrical changes. Sodium and potassium ions enter and leave the nerve during the different phases of conduction and this ionic migration takes place at the nodes of Ranvier, constrictions in the myelinated nerves at intervals of about 1 mm. The potential resulting from the migration of these ions extends from one node to another and thus the impulse passes along the nerve. Although the mechanism is not fully understood, local analgesic drugs stabilise the nodal membrane to prevent permeability to ions and this interferes with the passage of impulses along the nerve.

Local anaesthetic solutions are stored for injection as water-soluble salts, usually the hydrochloride. Such solutions are acid, having a low pH. When injected, they come in contact with tissues which are alkaline (having a pH about 7.4) and this is sufficient to cause a reaction which liberates the base of the local anaesthetic. If a solution is injected into an infected area where the pH is low—5.6 or less—the salt will fail to liberate base. This accounts for the failure of local analgesics to act in the presence of infection.

Topical application (Fig. 1.7)

Local analgesic solutions may be painted or sprayed on mucous membranes or wound surfaces. They are absorbed locally and produce analgesia of the area to which they have been applied. This method is not effective when the solution is applied to unbroken skin as the drug is not absorbed and does not reach the nerve endings.

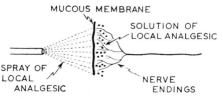

Fig. 1.7 Topical application.

Topical analgesia is used commonly for examinations or minor surgical procedures of the urethra, nose, throat and bronchial tree. In preparing a wound for cleansing and local infiltration, it may be of value to begin by using a swab which has been soaked in a dilute solution of a local analgesic.

Local infiltration (Fig. 1.8)

Injection of a dilute analgesic solution in the area of the proposed operation will block the perception of pain at the level of the nerve endings. This is perhaps the simplest method of analgesia and is used widely for minor surgical operations. If restricted to this type of case, it is a safe procedure and has few, if any, after effects so that the patient is able to eat and drink and return home shortly after the operation. The method can be used for more extensive operations but larger doses of the drug are necessary and side

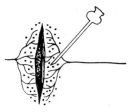

Fig. 1.8 Local infiltration.

effects are more likely. Extensive infiltration is also an unpleasant procedure for the patient. It is a common fallacy that local infiltration using dilute analgesic solutions is an entirely safe procedure. This is true only when two safeguards are observed. First, great care must be taken to avoid administering an overdose. It is easy to forget that in extensive procedures considerable quantities of the drug may have been injected, although in dilute solution. Local analgesic agents have toxic properties as have other drugs and an overdose may be lethal (see p. 205). In the second place, care must be taken to avoid intravascular injection of these drugs. Before and at intervals during the infiltration of the area of operation, aspiration with the syringe must be performed regularly to ensure that the needle does not lie within a blood vessel.

This technique is an excellent method for the surgeon working without the assistance of an anaesthetist. Provided the safeguards described are observed carefully, the technique is almost without complications. The method should not be used in the presence of local infection and is sometimes better avoided where the anatomy of the area may be distorted by the injection. This latter objection may be overcome by incorporating hyaluronidase in the solution.

Nerve block (Fig. 1.9)

The main nerve which supplies the area of an operation can be blocked by injecting a local analgesic solution close to it. Thus, it is possible, with a few injections, to produce analgesia for a wide area. This is achieved by using quite small doses of the drug and may be less harmful than widespread infiltration. The technique has the advantage that the solution may be injected some distance proximal to the site of operation so that distortion of the anatomy is avoided and the presence of sepsis at the operative site is not a contra-indication.

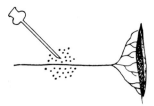

Fig. 1.9 Regional nerve block.

The technique is of particular value when the nerves which supply an area are easily accessible. With this method, as with those which follow, the presence of a bone structure which will act as a landmark in positioning the tip of the needle improves the chance of success. For example, the first rib is a convenient landmark in supraclavicular block of the brachial plexus (p. 212). In attempts to block the sciatic nerve, there are no bone structures immediately adjacent to the nerve and failure is more frequent.

Paravertebral nerve block (Fig. 1.10)

In this method, the nerves are blocked close to the vertebrae, before the sympathetic fibres have left the main nerve. This tech-

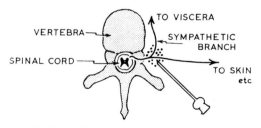

Fig. 1.10 Paravertebral nerve block.

nique can be used for surgical procedures inside the abdomen but, as it involves multiple injections, it is no longer popular for this type of case. Its use, therefore, is restricted to the blocking of a few nerves such as those innervating a leg, to produce vasodilatation in vascular disease.

We will now consider two techniques which, by one single injection, may produce analgesia over a wide area of the body.

Spinal or subarachnoid analgesia (Figs 1.11 and 1.12)

A local analgesic solution introduced into the cerebrospinal fluid may be distributed widely to affect a large number of nerves. In this way, by one injection, analgesia, muscular relaxation and sympathetic blockade affecting a large part of the body may be produced easily.

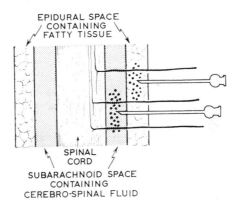

EPIDURAL SPACE
CONTAINING
FATTY TISSUE

SPINAL
CORD

SUBARACHNOID SPACE
CONTAINING
CEREBRO-SPINAL FLUID

Fig. 1.11 Epidural and spinal analgesia: the diagram illustrates the two sites at which the analgesic solution is deposited, following introduction of the needle through the intervertebral space.

The technique has many advantages:

1. Excellent analgesia results.
2. Muscular relaxation is complete.
3. Sympathetic blockade occurs. This produces not only a reduction in arterial pressure which may be advantageous in reducing haemorrhage at the operative site, but also a contracted bowel which allows easy access to all parts of the abdomen.
4. The volume of solution which will produce a given area of analgesia can be estimated readily.

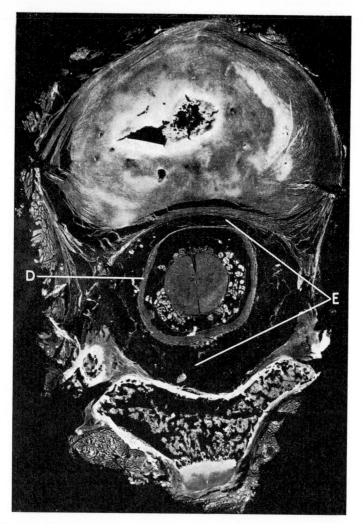

Fig. 1.12 Transverse section of spine between 1st and 2nd lumbar vertebrae. E is the epidural space and D the dura and arachnoid maters separating it from the subarachnoid space.

5. It is possible, though undesirable, for one person to perform the subarachnoid block and then perform the operation. This practice is both advantageous and fully justified in many of the developing countries.

A disadvantage of spinal anaesthesia is that most patients prefer to be asleep during the operation, particularly in countries in which the services of trained anaesthetic personnel is available easily. For this reason spinal nerve block may be performed for its special advantages although a light general anaesthetic is given also.

In the past, spinal analgesia has been associated with a number of complications; some, which are minor in character, such as transient nerve palsy and headache, are relatively common; others, though less common, are severe, for example paraplegia. Such complications have followed spinal analgesia, even when given by competent anaesthetists using what have been apparently impeccable techniques. While headache is a minor complication, in that it is never responsible for the patient's death, it may be severe and intractable and may last for several days, making the patient extremely miserable. The occasional occurrence of paraplegia reduces the patient to a pitiable state and has resulted in legal action being taken against the anaesthetists. The possibility of these complications has, at least in the United Kingdom, deterred many anaesthetists from using the technique more widely, although at present there is a renewed interest in its use.

The complications of spinal analgesia have been investigated widely. The headache may be a result of leakage of cerebrospinal fluid through the lumbar puncture and this can be minimised by using a fine needle (25 gauge). Paraplegia has been attributed to many causes: infection, trauma, chemical irritation or the use of unsuitable solutions.

Extradural or epidural analgesia (Figs 1.11 and 1.12)
Most of the advantages of spinal analgesia without some of the complications may be obtained by extradural or epidural analgesia (the terms are synonymous).

As they leave the subarachnoid space the nerves pass through the adjacent epidural space which is filled with fatty tissue and connects with the paravertebral spaces. By injecting analgesic solution into the epidural space, it is possible to obtain conditions identical to subarachnoid blockade, namely good analgesia, sympathetic blockade and good muscular relaxation. The risk of introducing infection into the subarachnoid space and the possibility of direct damage to the spinal cord is eliminated. In addition, because the arachnoid membrane is not punctured, headache is unlikely. The main disadvantages of the technique are that the epidural space is more difficult to identify than is the subarachnoid space, and the fat in it makes the spread of the solution less predictable. Thus the solution when injected may spread up or down the space or it may leak out to the paravertebral space. Therefore, for a given volume of solution, it is less easy to predict accurately how far up in the space the solution will spread and to what level analgesia will be produced. It should be pointed out also that paraplegia, although very rare, has followed the use of this technique. Despite this, it is preferred by many anaesthetists when subarachnoid anaesthesia might otherwise be indicated.

It is possible to pass a catheter into the extradural space and inject through it, at intervals, repeated doses of the analgesic solution. This enables analgesia to be continued into the post-operative period; by reducing post-operative pain, deep breathing is facilitated and post-operative chest complications may be reduced. This method is also valuable in providing pain relief during labour (see p. 193).

2

Drugs used in anaesthesia

INHALATION ANAESTHETICS

There are two groups: those which exist as *gases* at room temperature and which are stored at a high pressure in cylinders; and those which are *liquids* at room temperature and which require to be vaporised in a carrier gas. In making his choice of an inhalation anaesthetic, the anaesthetist is concerned principally with the following factors:

Solubility in tissues, particularly in the lipid phase. High lipid solubility signifies a prolonged uptake to equilibrium and a prolonged recovery.

MAC value. A high MAC value (see also p. 6) may limit the depth of unconsciousness which can be achieved with the drug, having regard to the need for oxygen at an alveolar pressure not less than 29 kPa (220 mmHg) and the presence of carbon dioxide 5.3 kPa (40 mmHg) and water vapour 6.2 kPa (47 mmHg).

Irritation of the respiratory tract will limit the ease with which anaesthesia can be induced.

Flammability and risk of explosion when mixed with oxygen. This will exclude the use of surgical diathermy and requires full anti-static design features in the anaesthetic and operating rooms.

Volatility. A substance with high boiling point will be difficult to vaporise.

Compatibility with chemicals used for absorbing carbon dioxide in a closed circuit system. Some substances may decompose to form poisonous products.

Effect on vital functions. In depressing the brain, most agents depress the respiratory centre also. Excessive respiratory depression causes hypoventilation of the lung alveoli with consequent retention of carbon dioxide in the tissues, and hypoxaemia.

Depression of the myocardium may result in an inadequate cardiac output.

Serious cardiac arrhythmia. This is more likely with some agents than with others. This risk may be enhanced in the presence of increased concentrations of *adrenaline,* either endogenous, for example as a result of hypoxia or hypercarbia, or injected in the course of the surgical procedure.

Other undesired effects such as involuntary movements during surgery, nausea, vomiting or shivering in the post-operative period.

Muscle relaxation. The extent to which anaesthesia with the agent will be accompanied by muscle relaxation, thus aiding surgical access.

Toxicity. Some agents may be associated with damage to organs such as the liver or kidney. Such effects may be either a direct effect of the drug itself or may result from the formation of metabolites of the drug molecule.

Cost.

Availability. If drugs are stored in cylinders, these must be transported from the factory to the hospital, and there may be difficulty in obtaining supplies in remote areas.

The anaesthetic gases

Nitrous oxide has been known for more than 200 years. It is sometimes called 'laughing gas' because one of its early uses was as a music hall entertainment. It is pleasant to inhale, non-irritant and has no adverse effects on the vital organs. It is neither flammable nor explosive when mixed with oxygen. It is compatible with the infiltration of adrenaline to the tissues.

Nitrous oxide is poorly soluble in the tissues and its MAC value is just in excess of 100 per cent of one atmosphere. Thus, anaesthesia without hypoxaemia is not possible with nitrous oxide alone, except in a hyperbaric environment. In spite of these apparent limitations, it is the most commonly used inhalation anaesthetic. Its poor solubility ensures a rapid onset of, and a speedy recovery from, its effects and the absence of side effects is of great value. It should be given with not less than 30 per cent of oxygen (see p. 23) and this mixture is often used as a carrier gas for a suitable volatile agent.

Consider the situation in which a patient is to receive halothane anaesthesia for the repair of a hernia. If halothane is the sole anaesthetic, vaporised in a mixture of air and oxygen, an equilibrium concentration of 0.8 to 1 per cent of halothane would be required. The use of 70 per cent nitrous oxide in the carrier gas (approximately 0.7 MAC) reduces the necessary halothane concentration to about 0.3 per cent. Since the side effects of halothane may be undesirable (see below), this reduced concentration is preferable.

Nitrous oxide is an excellent analgesic. Concentrations not exceeding 50 per cent in oxygen are used for the relief of pain in labour, in the post-operative period, in the intensive care unit, and in first aid.

Cyclopropane. MAC is 9.2 per cent of one atmosphere. Compared with nitrous oxide, the uptake and elimination to equilibrium is slower, although it is rapid in comparison with many of the volatile anaesthetics. Because a high initial concentration can be tolerated, it can be used to provide a rapid induction of anaesthesia which is valuable in children and in adult outpatients. The gas is non-irritant and is accepted easily by the patient.

The cardiac output and the arterial pressure are well maintained. Cyclopropane is considered by some anaesthetists to be of value for poor risk patients such as those with intestinal obstruction or haemorrhagic shock. However, cardiac arrhythmia may occur, especially in the presence of increased circulating adrenaline, either endogenous or injected. Cyclopropane is a powerful respiratory depressant and the retention of carbon dioxide aggravates the effects of the drug on the heart. It is associated commonly with nausea and vomiting in the immediate post-operative period. Because cyclopropane is expensive, it is given in a closed circuit (see Chapter III) usually as a mixture of 10 per cent of the gas in oxygen. The major disadvantage of cyclopropane is that with either oxygen or air it forms an explosive mixture. Cyclopropane is not used commonly and, in some hospitals, it is no longer available because of the risk of explosion.

Volatile anaesthetics

Halothane (Fluothane). Introduced in 1956, this is by far the most popular volatile anaesthetic. It is not irritant and is neither explosive nor flammable in mixtures with oxygen. MAC is 0.75 and the agent is highly soluble in the tissues. It is a very powerful agent with which very deep levels of anaesthesia can be achieved easily. Thus, it is a dangerous drug in the hands of the inexperienced.

Halothane depresses ventilation and the circulation, having a direct effect on the myocardium. The heart is slowed and ventricular extrasystoles may occur. Cardiac arrest has resulted from the injection of adrenaline to the tissues in patients receiving halothane. A reduction in arterial pressure accompanies halothane anaesthesia almost invariably, although this is regarded as an advantage in many operations since blood loss is reduced. Muscular relaxation can be produced, but normally only by giving high concentrations of the drug with resulting hypotension and respiratory depression; many anaesthetists would regard such deep anaesthesia with halothane as unacceptable in most situations. The uterus is relaxed and this may be of value in procedures for external version of the fetus. In operative delivery, however, there is a risk of excessive blood loss from a relaxed uterus and inhaled concentrations of 0.5 per cent halothane should not be exceeded. Similar considerations apply in operations for the removal of a retained placenta and for therapeutic abortion. Unlike nitrous oxide, halothane is a poor analgesic.

The recovery from halothane anaesthesia is usually pleasant and uneventful, although slower than the recovery from cyclopropane and nitrous oxide. Marked shivering may occur after exposure to the drug for more than half an hour. This may be troublesome, especially since it may cause a three- to four-fold increase in the patient's oxygen consumption. Although the absence of nausea or vomiting can never be guaranteed after any type of anaesthesia, it is not a particular consequence of halothane.

Halothane has been submitted to clinical and laboratory studies more frequently and more thoroughly than almost any other drug known to medical science. In spite of this, there remains an important controversy as to whether it is capable of causing damage to the liver. If so, the frequency of this event is very small indeed. Some authorities believe that an effect on the liver is a sensitivity response occurring only on a second or subsequent exposure to the drug, especially within one month of the previous exposure. Particular anxiety has been voiced in relation to the possible hepatotoxicity from the use of halothane in patients who receive several halothane anaesthetics in the presence of ionising radiations, for example in connection with the insertion of radium needles for the treatment of carcinoma of the uterine cervix.

Because of the danger to the patient from inadvertent high concentrations of halothane vapour, even for short periods, it is essential that the drug be administered from an accurate vaporiser. Halothane should be vaporised in not more than 70 per cent nitrous oxide in oxygen, 100 per cent oxygen (usually in a closed circuit), or in oxygen-enriched air.

Methoxyflurane (Penthrane) is a halogenated ether. Because it has a high boiling point (104.6°C), it is not possible to obtain a high concentration of vapour at room temperature. MAC is 0.16 per cent. The vapour is neither explosive nor flammable in oxygen. The agent is highly soluble in fat and thus the time for uptake to equilibrium and recovery is prolonged. The vapour is pleasant to breathe. Deep methoxyflurane anaesthesia causes moderate hypotension and an acceptable degree of muscle relaxation.

A small proportion of methoxyflurane is metabolised in the body, producing, among other products, free fluoride ions. If these ions accumulate as a result of prolonged exposure to the drug, there is an established risk of damage to the distal tubules of the kidney resulting in high-output renal failure.

Methoxyflurane is used occasionally as a supplement to nitrous oxide anaesthesia for prolonged operations and it is popular in some obstetric units as an inhalation analgesic for women in labour. For the latter purpose, a calibrated inhaler delivers 0.3–0.5 per cent methoxyflurane in air, which is breathed for only a few minutes at a time.

Enflurane (Ethrane), another fluorinated ether, has been in use in several countries for about 10 years, but only became available in the UK in 1977. MAC is 1.68 per cent. The vapour is pleasant to inhale and it is not flammable. The drug has no important effect on the cardiovascular system, except at deep levels of anaesthesia when, like halothane, enflurane may cause arterial hypotension. Occasionally, the drug causes involuntary muscular movements associated with an epileptiform EEG pattern. There are no after effects from these neurological side effects, but the drug is considered unsuitable for patients suffering from epilepsy.

Trichloroethylene (Trilene) is a useful inhalation analgesic when given in concentrations of 0.35–0.5 per cent and is employed in many labour wards. For many years, trichloroethylene has been used as an anaesthetic but usually as a supplement to nitrous oxide in patients who have been heavily sedated with narcotic analgesics. The problem with trichloroethylene as an anaesthetic is that cardiac arrhythmia is common as is a rapid shallow respiratory pattern (tachypnoea) which leads eventually to inefficient alveolar ventilation. The MAC value is 0.17 per cent but the undesirable side effects noted above supervene long before the brain equilibrates with this concentration.

Trichloroethylene should not be used in the presence of injected adrenaline lest dangerous arrhythmia supervene. It is not flammable in mixtures with oxygen but produces toxic by-products in the presence of soda lime.

Diethylether (ether) was the most widely used of the volatile anaesthetics for many years. In industrialised countries, it has been virtually abandoned except for occasional indications for its use in children. It is inexpensive and easily available, however, and these factors, coupled with the recognised safety of ether, make it an attractive drug in the less developed communities.

MAC is 1.9 per cent; the vapour is extremely irritant to breathe and bronchial and salivary secretions may be alarmingly copious, especially if atropine has not been given as a premedicant. Breath-holding, coughing and laryngeal spasm during the induction of ether anaesthesia call for skill in its administration. The drug is highly soluble in the tissues so that the induction tends to be prolonged. On the other hand, the risk of accidental overdose is remote. Ether stimulates the sympathetic nervous system and the cardiac output is well maintained. At deep levels of anaesthesia with ether, muscle relaxation is excellent. Nausea and vomiting are a common sequel to ether and may be protracted. Ether vapour is inflammable in mixtures with air and explosive when the concentration of oxygen exceeds that in air.

Chloroform has probably been one of the most controversial anaesthetic agents. It is a very powerful anaesthetic, is relatively non-irritant and deep anaesthesia may be produced fairly easily. However, it has serious effects on the cardiovascular system and has been responsible for cardiac arrest. It may cause vagal inhibition of the heart, ventricular fibrillation and has a direct depressant effect on the myocardium. Nausea and vomiting after chloroform anaesthesia may occur in as many as 50 per cent of patients, and liver damage of varying degree has been reported. In terms of its physical characteristics, chloroform is very similar to halothane. The protagonists of chloroform claim that used as halothane is now used, in known concentrations with adequate oxygenation, and by trained anaesthetists, it has much to commend it, being very much cheaper than halothane. However, in spite of such enthusiasm, chloroform is seldom used in anaesthetic practice nowadays.

Carbon dioxide and oxygen
Carbon Dioxide has anaesthetic properties of its own when used in concentrations in excess of 30 per cent, but it is not for this reason that it is used in anaesthetic practice. It is a respiratory

stimulant, normally increasing both the rate and depth of breathing when added to the gas mixtures inhaled. It may be added directly to the mixture, from a cylinder which is normally kept on the anaesthetic machine, or it may accumulate in the anaesthetic circuit by allowing rebreathing. Carbon dioxide should be used as a respiratory stimulant with caution, since an excess may stimulate the endogenous production of adrenaline. It should never be used when ventilatory depression is suspected, since carbon dioxide will have been retained already and additional quantities will only worsen the degree of depression.

Concentrations in the region of 5 per cent may be of value during induction of anaesthesia, particularly with diethylether or other irritant vapours, so that ventilation is stimulated and induction time reduced; during upper abdominal surgery in an attempt to relieve hiccough; at the end of a long operation where hyperventilation has been practised and it is anticipated that the tension of carbon dioxide in the blood is reduced.

Oxygen must be given in all anaesthetic techniques. If air is used as the carrier gas the concentration will be 21 per cent approximately but greater concentrations are normally desirable in an anaesthetic mixture.

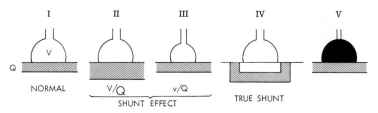

Fig. 2.1 Diagrammatic representation of shunt effect and true shunt within the lung. Example 1 shows the normal relation of ventilation to perfusion which will give optimum oxygenation of the blood in an air-breathing subject. Examples 2 and 3 represent regions of the lung in which perfusion is excessive in relation to ventilation. This will cause suboptimal oxygenation of blood unless the alveolar P_{O_2} is increased by increasing the inspired oxygen concentration. In examples 4 and 5 true shunt has occurred and the alveolar gas has no influence on the perfusing blood. Thus oxygen therapy will be of little use except that, by effecting an increase in the oxygen content of blood leaving the more normal alveolar units in other parts of the lung, the effect of a true shunt may be counteracted to a small extent.

During anaesthesia, either with the patient breathing spontaneously or where ventilation is controlled, oxygen transfer from the lung gas to the blood is impaired. A number of factors may cause this (Fig. 2.1), notably an alteration in the ventilation/perfusion ratio in the lungs (increased physiological 'shunt'), where perfusion is greatest in the dependent parts and ventilation is most effective in the upper zones. Depression of the cardiac output may lead to excessive desaturation of the blood returning to the lungs, the shunted fraction of this being mixed with normally oxygenated blood from the pulmonary capillaries. During controlled ventilation, unless large tidal volumes are used, some areas of the lungs may be underventilated leading to arterio-venous 'shunting' of blood.

While these mechanisms are complex, it should be stressed that the percentage of oxygen administered during anaesthesia should seldom be less than 30 per cent as this has been shown to compensate for the factors mentioned and to produce an arterial oxygen tension of at least 13.3 kPa (100 mmHg) in healthy subjects.

When suitable apparatus or supplies of nitrous oxide and oxygen are not readily available, the use of air as a carrier gas for a volatile agent such as halothane or ether has been recommended. While this technique has proved valuable, and in some circumstances will continue to be so, on the evidence quoted above its limitations must be borne in mind. The use of cyclopropane or halothane allows the administration of high concentrations up to 90 per cent of oxygen, and this method is practised by some anaesthetists.

There are possible adverse effects from breathing high concentrations of oxygen. Nitrogen is washed out from the alveoli and is replaced by oxygen; oxygen is absorbed rapidly and patchy collapse may occur. Further, by supplying excess oxygen with minimal respiratory effort, ventilation may become depressed in patients with chronic lung disease who exist normally on a 'hypoxic drive' to ventilation. Failure to recognise this problem in a spontaneously breathing anaesthetised subject may lead to respiratory arrest.

THE INTRAVENOUS ANAESTHETIC AGENTS

These include the intravenous induction agents and also a number of drugs given by intravenous injection which may be used alone or in combination with the inhalation anaesthetics to maintain anaesthesia during the operation.

The usefulness of an intravenous anaesthetic is determined by the following important factors:

Speed of onset of action. All of the drugs in regular use render the patient unconscious within seconds.

Speed of recovery. This may be rapid as in the case of some of the induction agents or prolonged as in the case of the narcotic analgesic, phenoperidine. A knowledge of the likely period of recovery will indicate the appropriate drug in a given situation.

Disposal in the body. If the drug is detoxicated or excreted rapidly, full recovery from its effects may be expected early. Alternatively, the drug may be given repeatedly with little risk of accumulation.

Quality of anaesthesia. Some drugs may produce sleep, although they are poor analgesics, while other drugs may have a profound analgesic effect but produce sleep only in very high doses. Anaesthesia induced by an intravenous anaesthetic may be associated with undesired side effects such as coughing, hiccough and involuntary movements.

The likelihood of depression of the cardiovascular system and the respiratory system. The 'therapeutic ratio' is the dose required to produce anaesthesia related to the dose which is associated with severe cardiovascular and respiratory depression.

Ease of administration. Some drugs may cause pain on injection and damage to veins, or tissue injury in the event of extravascular injection.

Convenience of preparation. Some compounds are stable in solution, while others have to be mixed immediately before administration.

Risk of hypersensitivity reactions.

Compatibility with other drugs likely to be administered during the anaesthetic.

Thiopentone sodium is the sulphur analogue of pentobarbitone. It it is supplied as a yellowish powder with an ampoule or bottle of sterile water sufficient to make a 2.5 per cent solution.* As the yellow powder contains 6 per cent sodium carbonate to stop the formation of the insoluble thiopentone acid, the solution has a high pH (10.4–10.6). This solution is prepared immediately before use as it is relatively unstable and is not normally kept for longer than 24 to 48 hours. Thiopentone, like other barbiturates, causes sedation and induces sleep but has no analgesic activity and it has been shown in small doses to have an anti-analgesic effect. This is

---

* In the past, 5 per cent solutions were available, but the consequences of intra-arterial or extravascular injection of such a high concentration are particularly serious and its use is not recommended.

responsible for some of the post-operative restlessness which is found in patients in whom anaesthesia has been induced with thio-pentone and in whom pain is a prominent feature. For this reason also, it is unsatisfactory to use thiopentone as the sole anaesthetic in any but the shortest procedures.

Thiopentone depresses the respiratory centre; after a deep breath or even a yawn, respiration is reduced, mainly in amplitude. Apnoea may supervene for a few moments then breathing restarts, shallow but regular. Surgical and other stimuli, such as vene-puncture, may increase the depth of breathing during this period.

A decrease in arterial pressure usually accompanies the injection of thiopentone, though this may be minimised by slow injection. It is largely a result of vasodilatation of the peripheral vascular bed and is transient, as a rule, provided only small doses of the drug have been given.

Another effect which is of importance is that the autonomic ner-vous system is depressed, the sympathetic more than the parasym-pathetic. This results in relative parasympathetic overactivity which may cause laryngeal spasm, bronchospasm, coughing and bucking during the induction of anaesthesia.

Recovery from a single 'sleep dose' of thiopentone is rapid, partly because of the breakdown of the drug in the liver, but mainly because of redistribution in the body. After recovery of consciousness, the redistributed drug is gradually returned to the blood and metabolised in the liver. Small quantities of barbiturate can be detected in the blood up to 24 hours after the administration of thiopentone and it is for this reason that it is dangerous for the outpatient to drive a car soon after apparent recovery or to con-sume other drugs, including alcohol. The breakdown products are excreted via the kidney and in patients with renal insufficiency the drug should be used with extreme caution.

The solution of thiopentone is extremely alkaline and if it is injected into the subcutaneous tissues or, worse, into an artery, severe damage may result. These complications are dealt with when considering intravenous induction of anaesthesia (p. 84).

Despite the introduction of many more modern intravenous anaesthetic agents, thiopentone is still the agent most widely used to induce anaesthesia.

Methohexitone sodium, a methylated oxybarbiturate, is one of the many drugs which have been introduced in an attempt to avoid some of the undesirable effects of thiopentone. It is used in 1 per cent solution which has a pH of 11.1. The time to both awakening and complete recovery is shorter than after thiopentone, and the patient wakens with very little 'hangover' effect. The outpatient, therefore, is able to leave the surgery sooner and more safely. Some patients who receive injections of methohexitone intravenously may complain of pain at the site of injection or along the course of the vein during the injection despite the fact that the needle is correctly positioned within the vein.

Some anaesthetists have found a high incidence of hiccough and of muscular movements and twitching following the administration of methohexitone. There is considerable disagreement as to how often this occurs, but it does so more often than after thiopentone. It may be that the incidence of muscular movement can be diminished by giving an analgesic premedicant such as pethidine. Many anaesthetists have found the drug useful in dental practice and in outpatient anaesthetic work, but so far it has not displaced thiopentone for routine use.

Althesin. In 1941, Hans Selye suggested that steroid molecules might be capable of inducing anaesthesia. The first compound to be employed commercially was hydroxydione which was a very successful anaesthetic having a duration of action of about 20 minutes, but its use was abandoned because of almost invariable thrombosis of the vein into which the drug had been injected.

Althesin is a mixture of two steroids, alphaxalone and alphadolone, in the proportion 3 to 1. It is prepared as an aqueous solution but cremophor EL, a derivative of castor oil, is required as a solubilising agent. Althesin is very satisfactory for inducing anaesthesia although it is not a powerful analgesic. Although it is capable of causing cardiovascular and respiratory depression, the therapeutic ratio is highly favourable. It is metabolised rapidly in the liver and there is little accumulation of the drug in the tissues. Attempts have been made to use Althesin as a continuous infusion, to provide anaesthesia without the use of gases, but even when drugs such as morphine and fentanyl have been added to the infusion to improve the quality of analgesia, the technique has enjoyed only limited success. Continuous infusions of Althesin have been used to provide long-term sedation or unconsciousness in patients undergoing controlled ventilation in intensive therapy units. The value of this technique is not yet clear.

Because Althesin is a mixture of substances, the dosage is usually expressed in millilitres. The average dose for the induction of anaesthesia is 0.05 to 0.1 ml per kg. This will provide about 10 minutes of light anaesthesia.

At the time of writing, Althesin is very popular as an intravenous injection agent in many countries. Nevertheless, there are reports of hypersensitivity reactions, the significance of which has to be regarded with caution. Improved methods of retrospective testing of patients who have exhibited hypersensitivity reactions, particularly by the immunologist, have suggested that while a few patients may indeed be sensitive to the steroid compounds in the vehicle, cremophor is suspect also. In addition, carefully conducted studies have suggested that other drugs which may be given at the same time as an intravenous induction agent, such as neuromuscular blocking drugs, may be the culprits on occasion. Moreover, it is not clear that Althesin is more likely to cause such reactions than are any of the other drugs which may be used as intravenous induction agents such as thiopentone. Neither the steroids in Althesin nor the earlier steroid, hydroxydione, have any hormonal activity.

Ketamine (Ketalar). This drug, a powerful analgesic, may be given to induce anaesthesia or to produce a state of dissociation short of unconsciousness with preservation of protective reflexes—particularly the laryngeal reflex. However, such protection is achieved only with small doses. The use of ketamine has been limited by the occurrence of systemic hypertension and a high incidence of vivid dreams or hallucinations during recovery; the latter may be prevented by the use of adequate sedative premedication. In addition, movement during operation may be troublesome in delicate surgery.

Nevertheless, in patients with bad facial burns, other conditions in which the airway may be difficult to maintain, and those undergoing cardiac catheterisation, the drug has been found useful. A tranquil recovery can be obtained by administration of diazepam before or towards the end of the procedure. Side effects appear to be less in children, in whom the drug finds its main applications. Because it does not depress the cardiac output, many anaesthetists regard ketamine as the induction agent of choice in the enfeebled patient, in those suffering from hypovolaemic shock and in those undergoing cardiac surgery.

The drug is administered in a dose range of 1–2 mg/kg by intravenous injection. It can be given by intramuscular injection when the dose is 10 mg/kg. Supplementary injections of ketamine can be used to prolong anaesthesia without the need to employ other agents.

Propanidid (Epontol). Propanidid, a non-barbiturate eugenol derivative, is an induction agent which enjoyed a brief vogue. The drug is approximately equipotent with thiopentone but is poorly soluble in water and is dissolved in an oily base with the aid of a solubilising agent cremophor EL; the solution is viscid. After the injection of a single dose of 5–7 mg/kg, the patient hyperventilates and loses consciousness for a period not usually exceeding 3–5 minutes. Recovery is more rapid and is complete earlier than after thiopentone. Propanidid is broken down rapidly without appreciable redistribution in the body. The drug potentiates the neuromuscular blocking action of suxamethonium but the incidence of post-operative muscle pains after suxamethonium is reduced.

Propanidid is extremely useful in outpatient anaesthesia but, because of anxiety about the risk of sensitivity reactions, some of which may have been a response to cremophor, its popularity has decreased.

Diazepam (Valium). This drug, a benzodiazepine, used principally as a tranquilliser, has been given by intravenous injection to induce anaesthesia. It is claimed that it produces less respiratory and circulatory depression than do the barbiturates. The results of intravenous injection are unpredictable, some patients being markedly affected by as little as 5 mg, while even large doses, 20 mg or more, may fail to produce unconsciousness although the patients readily accept an inhalation induction of anaesthesia. Injection of the drug is often associated with pain and subsequent thrombosis at the injection site. Diazepam has muscle relaxant properties; this effect, combined with the central depressant effect, make it valuable in controlling convulsions. It seems unlikely, however, that it will supplant the more established agents such as thiopentone for routine induction of anaesthesia.

Diazepam, or a related compound flunitrazepam, is most valuable for sedating patients who are undergoing surgery following a regional nerve block.

Neuroleptanalgesia

The drugs used in this technique comprise:

Neuroleptic drugs which produce a state of dissociation—usually a pleasant sensation but sometimes associated with acute anxiety. The best known is dehydrobenzperidol (droperidol). It is a potent anti-emetic agent, depressing the chemoreceptor trigger zone in the mid brain and has a mild adrenergic blocking effect which is thought by some to protect the peripheral circulation against the 'shock' of surgery. The dose is 5–10 mg for an average adult.

Unfortunately, it may also cause Parkinsonian tremors and delayed feelings of disorientation.

Potent analgesics: fentanyl and phenoperidine. Fentanyl (Sublimaze) is related chemically to pethidine and 0.1 mg is approximately equipotent with morphine 10 mg. The duration of analgesia with fentanyl is about 20–40 minutes. It shares with pethidine the ability to produce nausea and vomiting, cardiorespiratory depression and, in the long term, addiction. Phenoperidine (Operidine) has pharmacological effects very similar to those of fentanyl except that the duration of analgesia of 2 mg of the drug (= 10 mg of morphine) is about 90 minutes.

Mixtures of fentanyl with droperidol (Thalamonal) may be used to induce a state of unconsciousness with profound analgesia. Anaesthesia is maintained, thereafter, with nitrous oxide and oxygen and, when required, a muscle relaxant drug (see also p. 93). While it is claimed that a stable arterial pressure and some protection from shock is provided by the neuroleptanalgesic combination of drugs, it is the opinion of many that, apart from the duration of action of fentanyl and phenoperidine, the advantage of neuroleptanalgesia over the use of the more traditional analgesics such as morphine in the maintenance of anaesthesia is not striking.

THE PREMEDICANT AGENTS

The opiates. Although many sedative drugs are available, morphine and allied drugs are still widely used in premedication. They produce analgesia, psychic sedation and a state of euphoria which is very welcome before an operation. The opiates are non-irritant solutions and may be injected subcutaneously or intramuscularly. Their main disadvantages are that they produce a high incidence of post-operative vomiting, 30–40 per cent, and are respiratory depressants. In addition, they increase parasympathetic activity, predisposing to laryngeal spasm and possibly bronchospasm. It has been suggested that they should not be used in asthmatic patients for this reason.

Morphine sulphate is given normally in a dose of 0.15 mg/kg to a maximum of 15 mg. Papaveretum, containing morphine plus the other alkaloids of opium, is usually administered in a dose of 0.2 mg/kg to a maximum of 20 mg. Papaveretum is considered less liable to produce nausea and vomiting than morphine sulphate, although this view is perhaps doubtful. Many of the disadvantages of the opiates are found when a too large dose is given for a particular patient.

Pethidine hydrochloride was introduced as a substitute for morphine. Pethidine is a poorer sedative and produces less euphoria than the opiates. Given in equi-analgesic dosage, the side effects are probably similar to those found after the use of morphine, and the sedative properties are much less (morphine 10 mg = pethidine 60–65 mg).

Pethidine is claimed to have a relaxant effect on the bronchi and may be useful as an analgesic in the first stage of labour; it is widely used in obstetric practice for this purpose.

The use of narcotic analgesics in premedication is questioned frequently. It is claimed that when they are administered to pain-free anxious patients, they may not relieve anxiety but may produce a state of confusion. It is also claimed that if narcotics are omitted from premedication but given during or after anaesthesia, when the patient is in pain, the incidence of emetic sequelae is reduced. Thus, attention has been directed towards other groups of drugs.

The hypnotics. Barbiturate or other hypnotic drugs may usefully replace opiates in producing a tranquil state in the pain-free patient awaiting operation. Given early on the day of operation, a compound such as sodium amytal 120 mg will produce several hours of peaceful drowsiness in young and middle-aged adults. This allows more flexible timing of premedication. While these drugs are not analgesics, relief of anxiety frequently reduces the severity of post-operative pain and a reduction in the dosage of analgesics may be achieved. Alternatively, a smaller dose of an analgesic drug may be combined with a sedative drug as premedication. Thus, the quality of pre-operative sedation may be improved and post-operative sickness minimised.

The phenothiazines. These drugs like the hypnotics have been used to allay pre-operative anxiety. Many of the group have anti-emetic properties also. As in the case of the hypnotics, few phenothiazines have any analgesic properties but they may usefully be combined with a small dose of an analgesic. Pethidine and promethazine in combination with or without atropine or hyoscine (the Pamergan series) are used occasionally. In children trimeprazine syrup (Vallergan) 2–4 mg/kg given orally is used widely.

The phenothiazines may produce hypotension, particularly in combination with some of the inhalation anaesthetic agents, and post-operative drowsiness may be prolonged. These factors limit their usefulness.

The benzodiazepines. These drugs, including diazepam (Valium), are used in premedication, either orally or by injection, as they have been shown to possess specific anti-anxiety properties. Small doses of the drugs may be given from the time of admission to hospital until shortly before operation. Lorazepam (Ativan), which produces marked amnesia, has been used in a single oral dose of 2–4 mg several hours before operation. Lorazepam induces protracted amnesia and may, as in the case of diazepam, be of value for the sedation of patients undergoing regional nerveblock and those patients requiring prolonged sedation in the intensive care unit.

When using any of the non-analgesic sedatives, of which there are many, as premedication in patients undergoing operations known to produce considerable pain, two points must be remembered. A method must be found to subdue reflex activity during operation, for example by the addition of a volatile anaesthetic to the inhaled gas mixture, or the administration of an intravenous analgesic. It is also essential to anticipate post-operative pain and the intravenous injection of an analgesic towards the end of the operation should be considered. Alternatively, adequate arrangements must be available to ensure that post-operative analgesics are administered as soon as they are required. Otherwise, a patient may become restless and confused, as a result of pain. On the other hand, it has been shown that if the analgesics are not given as premedication (when pain relief is not required) but delayed until during or after operation, nausea and vomiting are much reduced.

Atropine and hyoscine. One or other of these drugs is often given before an anaesthetic to minimise the parasympathetic overactivity which may occur during the anaesthetic itself. While the use of non-irritant inhalation anaesthetics reduces the need for these belladonna derivatives, they are still used widely.

Atropine and hyoscine have some common actions. Both depress secretions from the salivary glands and from the mucous glands in the bronchial tree. In addition, they antagonise the muscarinic effect of acetylcholine. The pupil is dilated, the bronchial musculature is relaxed and a slight increase in respiratory dead-space may result. The tone and peristalsis in the alimentary tract are diminished.

The two drugs, however, differ in certain respects:

Atropine is more effective in blocking the muscarinic effects on the heart. Thus, mild tachycardia follows its administration and there is less effect on the heart rate of such drugs as neostigmine or halothane which would otherwise cause bradycardia. It has, however, no sedative effect and in fact increases the basal metabolic rate and stimulates the medulla oblongata and higher centres. The dose for an average adult is 0.6 mg.

Hyoscine (scopolamine) differs in that it produces a depression of the central nervous system causing drowsiness, sleep and amnesia. These effects are valuable in premedication but should be remembered when the drug is combined with an opiate or pethidine. The action on the heart and bronchial musculature is weaker than that of atropine; the heart may be slightly slowed after the administration of hyoscine. However, the drying effect of the drug is greater than that of atropine and this may prove valuable when irritant agents are employed.

Hyoscine has been shown to have a beneficial effect in reducing the incidence of travel sickness and of post-operative vomiting. The main disadvantage of the drug is that, particularly in older people, it may cause confusion and restlessness which may be very distressing for the patient and his attendants. The dose for an average adult is 0.4 mg.

MYONEURAL BLOCKING DRUGS

The term myoneural blocking drugs is ponderous but is strictly correct to distinguish drugs which block transmission at the neuromuscular junction and which are commonly called 'muscle relaxants' from other drugs such as diazepam which, by effects on internuncial neurones or elsewhere, may produce partial relaxation of muscle but of a lesser order than that necessary for surgical anaesthesia.

Tubocurarine (curare), introduced in 1942, was the earliest drug to be used as a muscle relaxant in anaesthesia. Nowadays there are many drugs to choose from and in comparing their value the anaesthetist will have special regard to the following factors:

The type of block. The majority of drugs act by competing with acetylcholine at the end-plate without causing depolarisation (Fig. 2.2); thus, they are classed as the non-depolarising drugs. Conversely, a molecule like suxamethonium causes depolarisation of the end-plate with contraction followed by relaxation of the muscle fibre.

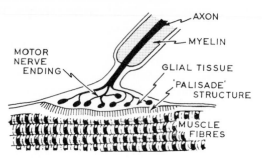

Fig. 2.2 The myoneural junction: the palisade structure is the site at which acetylcholine, released from the motor nerve endings, acts upon the muscle fibres to cause contraction.

Duration of action. A rapid onset of effect may be particularly important when there is a need for rapid tracheal intubation to secure the airway. A prolonged recovery may be inappropriate if the drug is being used for a short operation. Above all, however, predictability of the time of recovery is important.

Method of excretion or detoxication in the body. Gallamine, for example, is excreted by the kidney and would be contra-indicated in a patient with renal failure.

Ease of antagonism of the block following the administration of an anticholinesterase drug such as neostigmine.

Possibility of histamine release following injection.

Side-effects. Muscle relaxant drugs may mimic or block the effects of acetylcholine on other cholinergic receptors; thus they may produce ganglion blockade or parasympathomimetic effects.

Compatibility with other drugs which may be given in the course of anaesthesia including synergism and antagonism of the effects of either drug.

It must be stressed that the muscle relaxants have no analgesic or anaesthetic properties. It is essential therefore that the patient receives additional drugs to ensure analgesia and anaesthesia. Ventilation must be maintained by artificial means.

PHARMACOLOGY OF MUSCLE RELAXANT AGENTS

The competitive or non-depolarising relaxants

Tubocurarine. The South American Indians used curare as an arrow poison; their victims were paralysed and died from asphyxia. The drug is still refined from the extracts of plants brought from South America. It is administered in a solution containing 10 mg per ml and the average dose required to produce muscular relaxation, for abdominal surgery for example, is about 30 mg. Paralysis of all muscles develops in about 3 minutes and adequate time must be allowed for the drug to act. It is not preceded by stimulation of the muscles; there is a slow gradual cessation of activity of the respiratory muscles. In the dosage used in clinical practice (20–40 mg), few effects are seen apart from paralysis of the neuromuscular junction and a moderate reduction in arterial pressure. However, with larger doses and with normal doses in some individuals, ganglionic blockade may be caused and this is associated with a marked reduction in arterial pressure. It is also claimed that with the larger doses there may be histamine release and an asthmatic type of reaction may occur. These effects are rarely seen, however, and are not considered contra-indications to the use of the drug. A combination of halothane and tubo-curarine may be employed for their additive effects on the cardio-vascular system, producing profound but controllable arterial hypotension as a method of minimising blood loss during surgery (see p. 226).

Gallamine triethiodide (Flaxedil) is a synthetic agent which has an action similar to that of curare, though less potent (120 mg equal to about 30 mg of curare). In addition to producing paralysis at the neuromuscular junction, it causes tachycardia but has little or no effect on the arterial pressure and is less liable to produce histamine release than is curare. As a high percentage of the drug is excreted by the kidneys, its use is contra-indicated in the presence of impaired renal function. Because of tachycardia, it has been thought to cause excess bleeding during operation.

The effect of curare lasts from 30 to 40 minutes, while gallamine acts for 20 to 30 minutes.

Alcuronium (*Alloferin*) is about twice as potent as tubocurarine but has otherwise similar properties, although it does not release histamine from the tissues. The dose is 0.15 to 0.25 mg/kg. The duration of effect is about 25 minutes.

Pancuronium bromide (*Pavulon*) is five to six times more potent than tubocurarine. It is a very popular drug and a strong rival to tubocurarine in modern practice. It has little effect on the circulation, although mild hypertension and tachycardia have been reported occasionally. The dose is 0.08 mg/kg and the duration of action is about 45 minutes. Even a small overdose of pancuronium will cause a profound block which may be refractory to attempted antagonism with neostigmine. The drug is excreted in the urine, but a significant proportion is metabolised in the liver.

Fazadinium was introduced in 1976. As a clinically effective block may occur within 1 minute of injection, it has a more rapid onset of action as compared with the drugs listed above. The dose is 0.4 to 1.0 mg/kg. Its effect lasts for about 40 minutes. It is capable of both ganglion and parasympathetic blockade, and tachycardia may be troublesone. It is excreted in the urine and, as with gallamine, its use is not recommended in the presence of renal disease.

Antagonism of the non-depolarising relaxants
Neostigmine (Prostigmin), which is an anticholinesterase, allows the concentration of acetylcholine to increase and is an antagonist to the non-depolarising muscle relaxants. The dose for an adult is 2.5–5 mg.

The depolarising relaxants
Suxamethonium chloride (Scoline, Anectine) and suxethonium bromide (Brevidil E) have an action similar to that of acetylcholine. They produce initial muscle twitching and fasciculation followed by paralysis which lasts from 2 to 4 minutes. Following the administration of suxamethonium (0.6–1.2 mg/kg), there is a transient increase in arterial pressure and often a slowing of the heart rate which is particularly noticeable with second and subsequent injections of the drug. It has been reported that in some cases the heart has stopped for a period of up to 7 seconds. These effects can be minimised by the intravenous administration of atropine before the induction of anaesthesia. The administration of suxamethonium produces a transient small increase in the serum potassium concentration. This effect may be ignored in normal subjects but may be associated with dangerous cardiac arrhythmia and the possibility of arrest in patients with pre-existing hyperkalaemia or in the presence of gross tissue damage such as occurs in serious burn injury.

Suxamethonium and suxethonium are hydrolysed in the blood by pseudocholinesterase found in the plasma. In some cases, this enzyme may be atypical or may be abnormally low in concentration, and the effect of suxamethonium may be prolonged for a considerable period. There is no antagonist to these depolarising relaxants except reconstituted fresh frozen plasma which contains pseudocholinesterase. Under most circumstances, however, the lungs should be ventilated artificially until spontaneous recovery occurs. Even in the presence of a high concentration of abnormal enzymes, apnoea is unlikely to exceed 8 hours.

METABOLISM AND TOXICITY OF ANAESTHETICS

Until recently, it was believed that many of the gases and volatile agents were excreted unchanged by the body. Recent research suggests, however, that the hydrocarbon anaesthetic agents are metabolised to some extent, mainly in the liver. While the liver detoxifies many drugs, producing end products which are harmless or more easily excreted by the body, some anaesthetics may undergo biotransformation which results in metabolites which are more toxic than the original drugs. The role of fluoride in the renal toxicity of methoxyflurane is a good example which has been discussed previously.

Studies of pregnant rats and mice have demonstrated that prolonged exposure to any one of several inhalation anaesthetics may cause either shedding of the products of conception or fetal abnormality. On the basis of these findings, it is assumed that anaesthetics may be teratogenic in humans, and women who are, or who are likely to be, pregnant should not receive any of the general or local anaesthetic drugs during the first trimester unless they are to undergo surgery for a life-threatening condition such as acute appendicitis.

In addition, there is controversy as to whether the general anaesthetics are carcinogenic in some species. The air of operating rooms and recovery areas is usually contaminated by trace quantities of the gaseous anaesthetics and people who work in these parts of a hospital carry small amounts of the anaesthetics in their blood and other tissues. Several epidemiological studies have suggested that pregnant women anaesthetists and operating room nurses are more likely to suffer spontaneous abortion compared with control groups, while all such women may be more at risk from cancer. Because of fears that this may be a result of chronic exposure to anaesthetics, methods of disposal of gases exhaled from anaesthetic circuits should be employed. However, the risk from breathing contaminated air is by no means established. (See p. 50 for methods.)

Detoxification of a wide variety of drugs takes place in the liver by the microsomal enzyme systems. Severe liver disease or damage by drugs reduces the efficiency of these systems and a small dose of an opiate, for example, may exert an unexpectedly profound and prolonged effect.

Conversely, prolonged exposure to, or pre-treatment with certain drugs, notably phenobarbitone, but also alcohol and some of the volatile anaesthetics, results in enzyme induction. This means not only that increasing doses of these drugs may be required to produce the same effect, but, as the enzyme systems are non-specific, an unexpectedly poor response to a different drug may result from its over-rapid metabolism.

3

Anaesthetic machines and apparatus

The anaesthetic 'machine' is composed of four simple systems (Fig. 3.1):

1. A supply of compressed gases at a pressure of 413 kPa (60 lb/sq in)
2. A method of releasing and metering the gases
3. A method of vaporising volatile anaesthetic agents
4. A means of delivering the gases and vapours to the patient

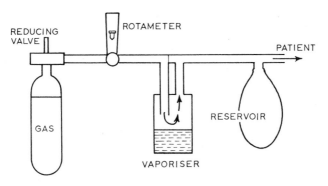

Fig. 3.1 Diagrammatic representation of the five components of a simple anaesthetic apparatus.

The supply of gases

This may take one of two forms. In modern hospitals, oxygen and nitrous oxide are each delivered by a supply pipe from a central source. Carbon dioxide and cyclopropane are delivered from cylinders mounted on the anaesthetic trolley. A reserve cylinder of oxygen and nitrous oxide should be maintained on each trolley in addition. In older hospitals, however, the supplies of nitrous oxide and oxygen may come exclusively from cylinders mounted on the trolley.

The cylinders are readily identifiable, each being painted in a distinctive colour:

Oxygen—black with white shoulders   Cyclopropane—orange
Nitrous oxide—blue   Carbon dioxide—grey

In addition, the name of the gas is printed on the cylinder as is the chemical symbol. A further safeguard against connecting a cylinder to the wrong inlet or valve is that in the head of the cylinder, beside the part from which the gas flows, two small holes are drilled in positions specific for each gas (Fig. 3.2). These match two pins on the reducing valve or pressure regulator (see p. 41).

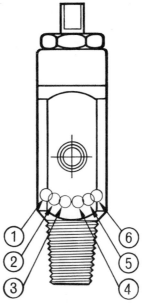

Fig. 3.2 This diagram shows how the holes on the cylinder neck are drilled on an arc. Only two holes are found on each cylinder, e.g.: 2 and 5 on oxygen cylinders, 3 and 5 on nitrous oxide cylinders, 3 and 6 on cyclopropane cylinders.

In addition to identifying cylinders, it is important to know how much gas each contains. In the case of oxygen, the reducing valve connected to the cylinder has attached to it a pressure gauge and the contents of the cylinder can be measured by estimating the pressure. A full cylinder contains gas at a pressure of approximately 13.8×10^6 Pa (2000 lb/sq in) and, as the volume of gas in the cylinder decreases, the pressure is reduced proportionately. Nitrous oxide and carbon dioxide are stored as liquids and the pressure above the liquid is little changed until there is no liquid remaining in the cylinder. Because of this, a pressure gauge on nitrous oxide and carbon dioxide cylinders does not indicate the extent to which the cylinder has emptied until approximately one-third of the contents remains. For such cylinders, the normal method of ascertaining how much gas remains is to weigh the cylinder and subtract the tare weight which is embossed on the neck (100 litre of nitrous oxide weighs 0.8 kg).

Most anaesthetic machines are equipped with a device which gives a visual and audible warning that the oxygen cylinder is empty. Clip-on labels are provided which should be attached to the cylinder or its outlet showing the words 'full', 'in use', or 'empty'. When a cylinder becomes empty, it should be removed as soon as possible and be replaced with a full cylinder, failing which an 'empty' label should be attached. If this is not possible, it is wise to disconnect the reducing valve from the cylinder as a reminder that this cylinder must be replaced at the first opportunity. It is dangerous to allow empty cylinders to remain attached to an anaesthetic trolley and it is many times more dangerous to commence using an apparatus without checking that the gas supplies are adequate.

Reducing valves (pressure regulators)

Pressures of the gases in cylinders vary from 48.3×10^5 to 138×10^6 Pa (700–2000 lb/sq in). Such pressures are not manageable when metering the gases through an anaesthetic machine and they must be reduced to workable levels. A pressure regulating valve is used for this purpose (Fig. 3.3). Each valve bears an identifying colour similar to that of the cylinder for which it is intended and it is also labelled with the name of the appropriate gas. At the point of attachment to the cylinder, there are pins which correspond to the holes drilled in the head of the cylinder. Since nitrous oxide and carbon dioxide are changing from the liquid to the gas phase, there is a large consumption of heat (the latent heat of vaporisation) and the pressure regulators for these gases have fluting on their outside surface to improve heat exchange with the atmosphere. Without such fluting, the pressure regulator might freeze and cease to function.

Flow meters

The flow meters in common use are known as Rotameters (the trade name of the largest manufacturer of these instruments). They consist of tapered glass tubes in which an aluminium bobbin spins (Fig. 3.4). The gas flow is indicated by the height of the top part of the bobbin and is read against the scale marked on the tube.

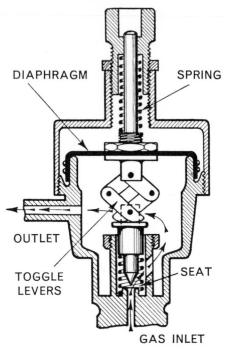

DIAPHRAGM   SPRING

OUTLET

TOGGLE
LEVERS   SEAT

GAS INLET

Fig. 3.3 Working principle of Adams' valve. When the outlet is occluded the pressure on the valve rises, the diaphragm lifts and the toggle levers force the pin into the valve seat, stopping the flow of gas from the cylinder.

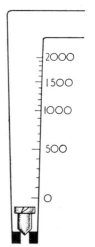

2000

1500

1000

500

0

Fig. 3.4 The Rotameter. As gas enters at the lower end the spinning bobbin rises in proportion to the flow of gas.

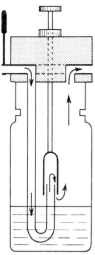

Fig. 3.5 A simple vaporiser—the Boyle's bottle. The arrows indicate the direction of gas flow.

Vaporisers

These are of two types. The simple vaporiser (Fig. 3.5) is suitable for vaporisation of trichloroethylene and diethylether where the exact concentration of vapour emitted is not critical. A lever at the side of the bottle directs an increasing amount of the gas into the bottle and when the plunger is depressed, the stream of gas coming from the 'J' tube is directed on to or through the fluid in the bottle.

Many factors govern the concentration of volatile anaesthetic given off from the simple vaporiser. Among these are:

— Ambient pressure and temperature
— Temperature and vapour pressure of the agent
— Rate of carrier gas flow through the vaporiser
— Area of the gas/liquid interface
— Position and movement of the vaporiser

The variations in these factors which may take place are quite considerable and are unacceptable when using a drug such as halothane or enflurane.

The vaporiser shown in Figure 3.6 compensates automatically for changes in the factors mentioned above and can deliver known concentrations of the vapour for which it has been designed in increments of 0.5 per cent. Similar vaporisers have been designed for use with other commonly used volatile anaesthetics, such as trichloroethylene and methoxyflurane. The effect of using ether in a simple vaporiser and a temperature compensated vaporiser is shown in Figure 3.7.

Delivery of the gases and vapours to the patient

Magill attachment (Fig. 3.8). This consists of a corrugated rubber tube, a reservoir bag, and a spill valve. The reservoir is necessary since the flow of gas from the machine is continuous during all phases of breathing whereas the patient's demand for these gases occurs only during inspiration. At the patient's end of the tube is placed the unidirectional spill valve (Heidbrink) through which excess gas may pass during expiration. The immediate connection to the patient is made with a mask, which is placed over the patient's face, or with a tracheal tube.

When using this type of circuit, it is necessary to deliver from the machine a flow of gases at least equal to the patient's alveolar minute volume (usually 5–6 litre/min), otherwise carbon dioxide will accumulate and will be rebreathed. The system should not

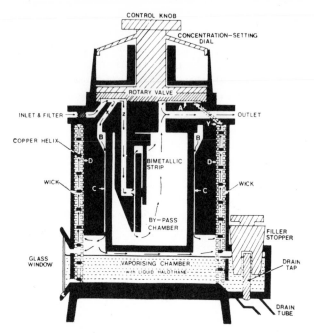

Fig. 3.6 The Fluotec Vaporiser Mark 3. This schematic diagram shows the construction of the vaporiser. The concentration-setting dial is in an 'ON' position. A = vapour control chamber; B = annular expansion chamber; C = long annular throat; D = spiral outlet channel of vaporising chamber; X = inlet to vaporising chamber; Y = outlet from vaporising chamber; Z = inlet to bypass chamber. (From Paterson, G. M., Hulands, G. H. & Nunn, J. F. (1969) *British Journal of Anaesthesia* 41, 109.)

be used for more than a few minutes if ventilation of the lungs is being controlled artificially.

A non-return or non-rebreathing valve (Fig. 3.9) may be used instead of the conventional Heidbrink valve. In this case, during expiration all the expired gas passes to the atmosphere and rebreathing of carbon dioxide is minimal.

The T-piece circuit (Fig. 3.10) introduced by Ayre is used in children when the resistance to expiration offered by valves is harmful to the child, particularly if spontaneous breathing is to occur for a prolonged period. The open limb of the T-piece conveys expired gas to the atmosphere and acts as a reservoir.

The closed circuit. In the closed circuit (Fig. 3.11), the patient's expired gas passes through 'soda lime' (a mixture of calcium hydroxide 95 per cent, and sodium hydroxide 5 per cent) which

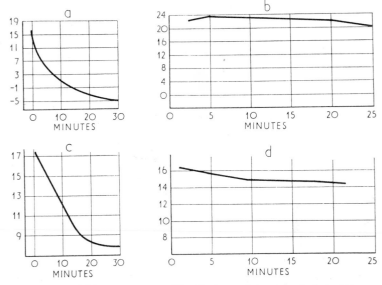

Fig. 3.7 The fall in temperature of liquid ether and decrease of ether vapour concentration in the output, when comparable gas flows are passed through a Boyle's bottle and a temperature compensated vaporiser. (a) Temperature change with time in Boyle's bottle (°C). (b) Minimal temperature change with time in a compensated vaporiser (°C). (c) Ether concentration change with time from a Boyle's bottle (vol. %). (d) Fairly constant ether concentration leaving a compensated vaporiser over a period of time (vol. %).

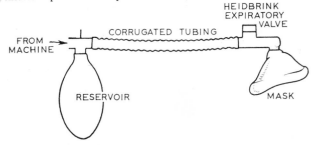

Fig. 3.8 The Magill attachment.

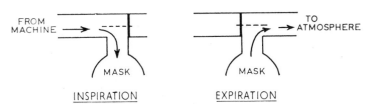

Fig. 3.9 A non-return valve. During inspiration the valve slides across and permits the patient to breathe gases from the machine. On expiration the valve cuts off the supply of gases from the machine and allows the expired gas from the patient to pass to the atmosphere.

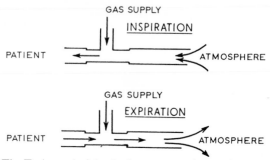

Fig. 3.10 The T-piece principle. As there are no valves, resistance is minimal and, by adjusting the flow of gases and the length of the expiratory limb to the atmosphere, the degree of rebreathing can be controlled.

absorbs carbon dioxide almost completely. The gas then passes to the reservoir bag and can be used again, provided that a small quantity of oxygen equal to the metabolic consumption of the patient (approximately 250 ml/min) is added to the circuit. Such a system offers several advantages:

— Economy of gases and vapours
— Conservation of moisture and heat
— Avoidance of contamination of the theatre atmosphere with anaesthetic gases
— A reduction in the risk of explosion when inflammable agents are being used.

However, extra rubber tubing is required and valves must be interposed to keep the gases flowing in the correct direction. In

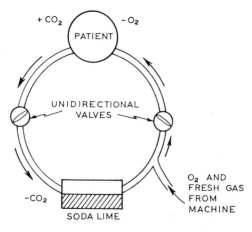

Fig. 3.11 Diagram of a closed circuit circle absorption system.

addition, the use of soda lime further increases the resistance to spontaneous breathing. During controlled ventilation, this increase in resistance is less important since the work of breathing is undertaken by the anaesthetist or a machine. Trichloroethylene must not be used in association with soda lime since it decomposes to form toxic products. The increased resistance to breathing in a closed circuit is usually unacceptable for children.

Many anaesthetists, particularly in North America, use the 'closed circuit' with a flow of gases greater than the basal oxygen requirements. This means that a spill valve in the circuit must be open and that there is considerable spillage from the circuit to the operating theatre environment. This is less economical than

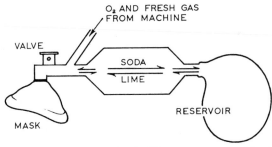

Fig. 3.12 The Waters anaesthetic circuit. The gases pass to and fro through the soda lime canister.

a completely closed circuit but it minimises the chance of a dangerous concentration of gas or vapour being built up and is said to be more efficient in ensuring the removal of carbon dioxide than is reliance on the absorber alone.

In addition to the type of closed circuit system illustrated in Figure 3.11, it is possible to use an alternative arrangement in which the gases pass through the soda lime both in inspiration and expiration (Fig. 3.12). This arrangement is known as Water's circuit, and is less popular than previously, largely because the soda lime canister which is heavy must be positioned close to the patient and may be difficult to position without causing traction on the face mask or endotracheal tube.

Intermittent flow machines

Most of the anaesthetic machines are based on the continuous flow principle, that is, the fresh gas flows to the circuit at a constant rate throughout all phases of breathing, the excess during expiration being accommodated in a reservoir. Other systems, such as the Walton apparatus for dental anaesthesia, and the Entonox

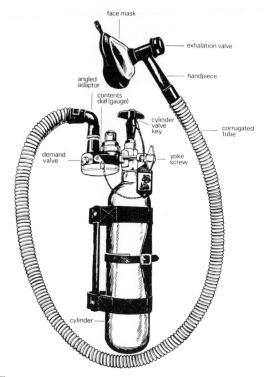

Fig. 3.13 Entonox apparatus for self-administered 50 per cent nitrous oxide in oxygen. The gas leaves the cylinder only when the patient makes an inspiratory effort.

(pre-mixed 50 per cent nitrous oxide in oxygen) analgesia apparatus supply gases to a patient only in response to the patient's inspiratory effort (Fig. 3.13). It is essential to ensure a gas-tight fit between the patient's face and the mask, or the system will not function satisfactorily.

Other methods of administration

The open mask
The Schimmelbusch mask (Fig. 3.14), originally introduced for use with chloroform, consists of a base with a frame over which a layer of lint is placed. The shape of the frame does not allow a gas-tight fit and thus air or oxygen can be drawn in between the face and the mask. It may also be used to administer diethyl-ether to small children. The Ogston mask is superior for the administration of ether (Fig. 3.15). Several layers of gauze are placed

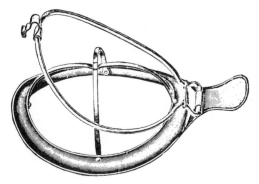

Fig. 3.14 Schimmelbusch's mask.

over the frame and a towel is pinned round the built-up portion to ensure that some of the vapour is retained above the gauze and reinhaled along with accumulated carbon dioxide, which acts as a respiratory stimulant. In addition, a gas-tight fit is obtained by placing over the face a gamgee pad with a hole cut in it, through which the patient breathes. This ensures that all inspiration and expiration takes place through the gauze.

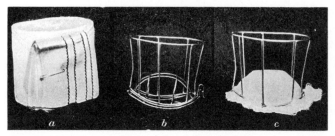

Fig. 3.15 Ogston's ether inhaler. (a) Inhaler fully draped and ready for use. (b) Frame of inhaler. (c) Inhaler with gauze only, but before towel is pinned round uprights.

Draw-over vaporisers
While open masks have the advantage of portability, many of their disadvantages can be overcome by using a draw-over vaporiser such as the EMO temperature compensated ether draw-over vaporiser (Fig. 3.16). The patient inhales atmospheric air through the vaporising chamber, and the design ensures that the inspired concentration of ether is known accurately. The bellows system, shown on the left of the figure, acts as a reservoir and also as a method of monitoring breathing. If the anaesthetist wishes to control ventilation, manual compression of the bellows provides a

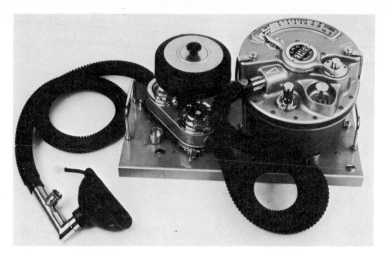

Fig. 3.16 Emo apparatus.

source of gas under positive pressure. This system can be used to control ventilation in a patient who has received a myoneural blocking drug; 3–4 per cent of ether in air will be sufficient to provide an anaesthetising gas mixture under these circumstances.

Where there is a need to enrich the oxygen content of the inspired gas, oxygen from a cylinder can be admitted through a port incorporated in the bellows system.

Trichloroethylene in air is used commonly as an analgesic in obstetric practice. Draw-over vaporisers for this purpose, such as the Emotril and Tecota systems, deliver accurate concentrations of trichloroethylene (0.35 or 0.5 per cent) in air to the patient.

CONTAMINATION OF THEATRE AIR

The removal of exhaust gases is now regarded as an important safeguard of the health of operating theatre personnel. There are two methods in common use:

Passive. The gases are led outside the hospital building via a copper conduit. The flow along the conduit is caused by the patient's expiratory effort. This method is simple and inexpensive, but care must be taken to ensure that the resistance to flow is not excessive and that condensed water vapour is not accumulating in the conduit with the risk of retrograde flow to the patient's circuit.

Active. The gases are led to a reservoir, on the anaesthetic trolley, from which a pump carries them through a narrow-bore tube to the outside of the building. Such systems are expensive to install but are safer than the passive systems and are essential if the operating suite is situated at some distance from the outside walls of the building.

4

Pre-anaesthetic examination and therapy including premedication

Anaesthetic outpatient clinic
Ideally, all patients should be seen at an anaesthetic outpatient clinic at about the time that they are seen at the surgical outpatient clinic. This enables many conditions requiring treatment, such as anaemia, chronic bronchitis and dental sepsis, to be detected before the patient is admitted to hospital, thus saving time and beds. In some hospitals, all patients requiring surgery are referred to the anaesthetist, while in others only patients whose condition seems likely to require pre-operative therapy are referred for this purpose. In other hospitals, the anaesthetist may attend the surgical outpatient clinic.

Few hospitals have such facilities, however, and in most cases the examination and treatment of patients in the pre-anaesthetic period takes place after admission to hospital for surgery.

PRE-ANAESTHETIC EXAMINATION

The object of this examination is to detect any abnormality which will increase the risks of surgery and anaesthesia.

History
Special attention is paid to the following:

Mode of life. The patient's occupation and his habit as regards exercise, alcohol and tobacco.

Previous illnesses. Especially those which may have left some damage, for example rheumatic fever or diphtheria.

Note is taken of any history of asthma or other allergic disease, and other more unusual conditions such as porphyria.

Drug therapy. Details are sought of any drugs which the patient is taking or has been taking during the previous two years. Specially important are steroids, sedatives and drugs affecting the cardiovascular system, particularly antihypertensive drugs.

Previous anaesthetic experiences. Note any complications which have occurred in the patient and his blood relatives, and the personal preferences of each patient for individual techniques.

Surgical condition for which the operation is proposed. Elicit any symptoms or signs which may be relevant to the anaesthetic, for example a patient who has been bleeding copiously will be anaemic.

Symptoms suggestive of cardiorespiratory insufficiency or disease. Questions are directed to symptoms such as cough, breathlessness on exertion and swelling of the ankles.

While taking the history, the anaesthetist has an opportunity to assess the patient's nervous temperament and this will give him some guide in prescribing pre-operative sedation.

Respiratory system. While the patient's history regarding cough, breathlessness on exertion and his degree of exercise tolerance are of considerable importance in assessing fitness for anaesthesia, routine clinical examination is equally important. Chest radiography should be performed in all patients undergoing major surgery. Where the history or examination indicates limitation of function or of exercise tolerance, special respiratory function tests may be carried out. These are discussed separately (p. 65). The haemoglobin concentration should be measured.

Cardiovascular system. Again the patient's history is important. The heart should be examined clinically and the arterial pressure measured. Where indicated, electrocardiography and other special tests may be performed (p. 63).

Urinary system. The urine is examined chemically and microscopically for any abnormal constituents such as sugar, albumen, blood or cells. Where any of these is present, further investigation of the urinary tract is undertaken. In many cases, particularly those patients undergoing major surgery, the blood urea concentration is measured.

Nutrition and hydration. In most patients admitted for elective surgery, little abnormality will be noted in this respect but in patients who have been suffering from wasting diseases or who have been vomiting or losing fluids from fistulae, it is important that blood should be sent for measurement of the plasma proteins, electrolytes, liver function tests and acid–base indices.

The system to be operated on should be examined if this is likely to have a particular bearing on the anaesthetic.

The nose, throat and teeth should be examined carefully for signs of deformity or infection which may influence the maintenance of an airway. In addition, the superficial veins should be examined carefully. Where it is intended to use a regional analgesic technique, the area of the contemplated injection should be studied carefully lest there are contra-indications to the use of such a technique.

Having examined the patient fully, the overall picture of his physical status may be established. The American Society of Anesthesiologists classifies physical status in the pre-operative period as follows:

Class 1   A normal healthy patient.
Class 2   A patient with mild systemic disease.
Class 3   A patient with a severe systemic disease that limits activity but is not incapacitating.
Class 4   A patient with an incapacitating system disease that is a constant threat to life.
Class 5   A moribund patient not expected to survive 24 hours with or without operation.

This method of grading the patient is often helpful in impressing on all concerned the necessity for energetic pre-operative treatment or, occasionally, for postponing operative treatment.

PREPARATION FOR ANAESTHESIA AND OPERATION

Treatment of established lesions
Where the patient has an acute respiratory infection, operation should be postponed if possible. The likelihood of post-operative chest complications is greatest when an anaesthetic is given during the first 3 to 4 days of a common cold, the so-called invasive period. If the operation cannot be delayed, an antibiotic may be given to reduce the danger of secondary bacterial invasion.

Patients with a chronic respiratory condition should, where possible, be operated upon during a period of remission, normally in the spring and summer. Physiotherapy, in the form of breathing exercises, should be given before operation and may be combined with the use of broncho-dilator drugs. The arterial blood gas tensions and the acid–base parameters should be measured as a baseline for post-operative therapy.

When the patient is found to be anaemic, it may be possible to institute iron therapy with a view to readmission to hospital later when the haemoglobin concentration has reached acceptable levels. If this is not possible, the patient may be given blood or, preferably, concentrated red cells, and a period of 3 days is allowed to elapse before the operation; it has been shown that transfused blood does not reach its maximum oxygen-carrying capacity in the first 2 days following transfusion. Elective surgery should seldom be undertaken where the haemoglobin concentration is less than 10 g/dl. Patients with long-standing anaemia are able to tolerate a reduced level of haemoglobin better than those who have become acutely anaemic. This tolerance is a result of altered 2,3-diphosphoglycerate concentration in the red cells with a favourable shift in the oxyhaemoglobin dissociation curve to the right.

The presence of mild uncomplicated arterial hypertension is not regarded as a contra-indication to anaesthesia. In many patients, it may be a sign of pre-operative anxiety and a second pre-operative assessment may reveal a value within the normal limits. If in doubt, selected cases may be treated by rest in bed and mild sedation for a few days.

More severe hypertension presents a difficult problem. It is now accepted that such patients benefit from anti-hypertensive therapy adjusted as necessary for the period of operation. Where possible, operation may be postponed until the patient has been established on a suitable antihypertensive regimen.

Cardiac decompensation will necessitate active treatment with digitalis, diuretics and other appropriate measures.

Diabetes. Patients who are receiving treatment with long-acting insulin or with oral hypoglycaemic agents, especially chlorpropamide which has a long half-life, should be brought under control with soluble insulin on the day before operation. On the day of operation itself, a glucose infusion is given. *Never give glucose orally before operation.* The urine is tested with one of the commercial colour indicator papers and insulin is given on the following sliding scale:

Colour	Treatment
Green	10 units of soluble insulin
Yellow	20 units of soluble insulin
Orange	30 units of soluble insulin

Each dose of soluble insulin is given subcutaneously. After operation, the regimen is continued, the urine being tested three-hourly and only when the patient is stabilised on diet are the long-acting agents recommenced.

Patients who have received steroid therapy should be considered as special anaesthetic risks. Anaesthesia, surgery and post-operative complications are considerable stresses for which the patient may be unable to compensate and this must be allowed for when pre-scribing supplementary steroid therapy. If there is any doubt about the competence of the adrenal cortex, the extent to which a patient is able to respond to stress may be determined by measuring plasma cortisol levels before and after the injection of ACTH.

Many patients may be receiving sedative therapy. These drugs may affect the course of anaesthesia in one of two ways. Patients who are receiving phenothiazine derivatives such as chlorpromazine may require very little thiopentone and, indeed, if more than minimal doses of this drug are given, marked arterial hypotension and prolonged recovery may follow. On the other hand, patients who are habituated to barbiturates or to alcohol may be very resistant to normal doses of anaesthetic agents and induction may prove difficult in such cases. This is the result of enzyme induction in the liver which results in excessively rapid breakdown of the anaesthetic agents.

The monoamine oxidase inhibitor group of drugs used in the treatment of depression may cause severe hypertension, particularly after amphetamine-like drugs. Abnormal reactions to narcotics, such as hypotension, hypertension and hyperpyrexia, may occur also. Such drugs may be associated with delayed recovery of consciousness after general anaesthesia and with liver damage.

Antihypertensive agents. Patients receiving such therapy present a problem to the anaesthetist. If such a patient is anaesthetised, a profound reduction in arterial pressure which may not respond to vasopressor therapy may be encountered. If, on the other hand, hypotensive therapy is discontinued, the patient is submitted to surgery with an increased strain on his myocardium, a reduced blood volume (because of peripheral vasoconstriction), and the risks from these states are added to the operative risk. A detailed discussion of the indications for continuing or discontinuing antihypertensive agents is beyond the scope of this book. Special mention should be made of methyldopa (Aldomet), which in our experience is the most commonly used antihypertensive agent at present. As this drug is unlikely to have interfered with the drugs which will be used during anaesthesia and with the resuscitative measures likely to be employed, the present recommendation is that it should not be discontinued in anticipation of anaesthesia and surgery.

Many patients who are being treated for hypertension may be receiving diuretics and this may result in potassium depletion with alteration in the response to myoneural blocking drugs. It is important to measure the serum potassium concentration before operation.

Beta adrenergic blocking drugs (propranolol, practolol). These drugs are employed in the treatment of a variety of conditions, notably in patients with angina. There has been considerable controversy about the advisability of continuing this therapy in patients undergoing anaesthesia and surgery. The current view is that therapy should be maintained, but there is increasing awareness that β-blockers may compromise circulatory compensation, particularly in the presence of hypovolaemia, when artificial ventilation is instituted. Additionally, in the unfortunate event of cardiac arrest, some anaesthetists believe that in the presence of beta blockade, there is greater difficulty in restoring the heart to sinus rhythm. For these reasons, attitudes to the continuation of beta blockade surgery may have to be reconsidered.

Antibiotics in large doses may potentiate the curariform drugs. All 'mycin' drugs such as neomycin and streptomycin are particularly important in this respect.

Oral contraceptives may inhibit the breakdown of pethidine in the body. Although they may increase the incidence of venous thrombosis during and after operation, current opinion is opposed to stopping therapy on the grounds that the adverse effects may take many weeks to disappear. Subcutaneous heparin therapy (5000 units) should be employed to reduce the risk of thrombosis.

Where examination reveals alteration in the plasma proteins or unsatisfactory electrolyte concentrations, intravenous therapy should be commenced to ensure that these deficiencies are remedied before anaesthesia and operation.

The purpose of the operation should be explained to the patient or his parent and *written permission for anaesthesia must always be obtained.* In Britain, an individual of 16 years of age or more may give consent for treatment without the authority of a parent or guardian, provided he is capable of understanding what the treatment involves. The consent of a parent or guardian should be obtained, however, when the patient is under 16 years of age. In an emergency, every reasonable effort should be made to obtain written consent but if the patient is unconscious, for example, or relatives are not readily available, essential treatment should not be withheld. The consent form should be kept in the patient's record folder and be checked by the anaesthetist.

Routine preparation

It is essential to ensure that every patient goes to theatre with an empty stomach. Of the small number of deaths each year which may be attributed to anaesthesia, one in every eight is a result of vomiting or regurgitating during anaesthesia. All these deaths must be regarded as preventable. Normally, no food or fluid is given to the patient by mouth for a period of at least four hours before operation. In addition, it is essential to ensure that the patient knows why this is being done and to ensure that he does not eat or drink from stores in his locker.

It may not be possible to observe the period of fasting when an emergency operation has to be undertaken shortly after a meal has been ingested. Also a four-hour period of fasting may not constitute a guarantee that the stomach is empty in conditions where the stomach fills up from below, for example in intestinal obstruction, or when emptying of the stomach is delayed notably following injury. In the past, many remedies have been advocated to deal with the problem of the full stomach or the more sinister sequelae. These include forced emesis, aspiration through a wide-bore tube and the insertion of blockers to occlude the outlet from the stomach. None of these measures can be recommended, however, although it is of importance to consider the use of antacid therapy to neutralise gastric acidity. Mist. magnesium trisilicate B.P. 15 ml may be given. The purpose of such treatment is to ensure that in the event of aspiration of gastric contents to the lungs, the material will be less acid, thus reducing the risk of aspiration pneumonitis. In the injured patient, metoclopramide (Maxolon) 10 to 20 mg i.v. may facilitate gastric emptying to the small bowel.

The bladder and bowel should be emptied. Where major bowel surgery is contemplated, enemata may have been given and some patients, particularly those undergoing gynaecological or urological surgery, will have a urethral catheter in place before operation or shortly after anaesthesia has been induced. It is essential to ensure that the outpatient undergoing light anaesthesia for the minor operation has the opportunity to empty his bladder and bowel lest he soil himself during the operation.

Artificial teeth, contact lenses, rings, hairpins and other objects liable to harm the patient should be removed.

PREMEDICATION OR PRE-ANAESTHETIC MEDICATION

Premedication may be given for three reasons:

1. To relieve anxiety. This may include pain relief
2. To abolish or reduce undesirable parasympathetic activity
3. To reduce post-operative vomiting

The relief of anxiety (sedation) is the most important function of premedication. When pain is present before operation, anxiety may be relieved by alleviating the pain. In other cases, psychic sedation is required.

Reassurance and simple explanations to the patient can save much in the way of drugs. Many patients will benefit from a simple explanation of hospital routine. They will appreciate being told that on the night before operation they will receive a hypnotic. They will also appreciate being told that, before going to theatre, pre-anaesthetic sedatives will be given so that they will approach the anaesthetic room with minimal anxiety. Many who have had previous surgery and have unpleasant memories of an inhalation induction will appreciate the promise of an intravenous induction. Despite the advent of medical television programmes, many patients know little of the routine of a surgical ward or theatre and their greatest fear is of the unknown.

While this psychological preparation is helpful, it is seldom in itself adequate to relieve anxiety and some form of sedative drug is normally given (see p. 30).

In very nervous patients, a mild sedative may be given for a few days before admission or soon after admission.

Parasympathetic overactivity during anaesthesia may be manifest as bradycardia, excessive secretion of saliva and bronchial mucus, or as broncho-constriction. Although, with the use of modern agents, irritation of the bronchi with excessive secretion is less common, and the routine use of a belladonna derivative is now being questioned, many anaesthetists still include such a drug in a premedicant mixture. The drugs used commonly are atropine sulphate or hyoscine hydrobromide (Scopolamine).

Atropine in appropriate dosage may be given to patients of all ages but has no sedative properties. *Hyoscine* provides welcome amnesia, the patient remembering little of what has happened. Its disadvantages are that it has no vagolytic action and, indeed, may cause slight slowing of the heart. In older patients, hyoscine may cause restlessness and confusion and its use is usually restricted to patients under the age of 60.

Often, atropine or hyoscine is incorporated in the premedication given about one hour before surgery. However, some anaesthetists, to avoid causing the patient to have a dry mouth during this period, omit the belladonna derivative from the original injection and inject it intravenously at the time of induction.

Post-operative vomiting has many causes but its frequency may be reduced by the use of appropriate drugs in premedication, such as hyoscine, the phenothiazines, cyclizine, droperidol or metoclopramide. They may be given alone or in combination with other drugs.

Timing and administration of premedication

The opiates and atropine are non-irritant solutions and may be given subcutaneously about 1 to $1\frac{1}{2}$ hours before operation. Many of the other drugs used, such as pethidine and the phenothiazines, are more irritant and are normally given by intramuscular injection 30 to 40 minutes before operation. This route should be used also if the patient is obese or if a rapid effect is required. It is useless and may be dangerous to give premedication at a time when it cannot possibly be absorbed before the induction of anaesthesia. Not only does the patient gain no benefit from the sedatives incorporated in it but these drugs will exert their maximum depressant activity during anaesthesia when depression from other agents is already maximal. If for any reason the injections have not been given at the prescribed time intervals, the drugs should be withheld and given intravenously by the anaesthetist.

Oral premedication

Oral premedication is attractive, particularly in children, because it avoids the unpleasantness of an injection. On the other hand, absorption from the stomach may be more variable than absorption from an intramuscular depot. Diazepam 10–15 mg by mouth for an adult of average size is an extremely popular method of sedation in current practice. Lorezapam (Ativan) is a related compound which is gaining popularity. The equivalent dose is 2.5–4 mg. As a rule, anaesthetists who use these drugs by the oral route are among those who do not consider than an anticholinergic drug is necessary in premedication. Sometimes, however, they accept that atropine may be given intravenously at the time of the induction of anaesthesia. In children, trimeprazine (Vallergan) syrup is given frequently.

In the past, the barbiturates and various hypnotics such as methaqualone (Mandrax) were popular in premedication, although the frequency of their use is diminishing. All the substances which have been described in this section are non-analgesic preparations. They have an important advantage, however, in that they are effective for a period of up to four hours or more after administration so that the timing of oral premedication is less critical than is the timing of premedicant drugs given by the parenteral routes.

After premedication has been given, the patient should be left in quiet surroundings so that it may take effect. In some units, the beds are screened-off for this purpose. Preparations such as the clothing of the patient in a theatre gown should be complete before premedication. Patients should not be allowed out of bed after premedication lest they feel dizzy and sick. The patient should be moved to the trolley to take him to theatre, gently and calmly.

Identification of patients

It is vitally important that all patients going to the operating theatre should bear adequate means of identification. This is becoming ever more important in view of the increasing work load falling on units which may be short of staff. The possibility of operating on the wrong patient or carrying out the wrong operation is increased under these circumstances. Identification is usually accomplished by attaching to the patient's wrist a label which bears his name, age, address and hospital number. Ideally, this label should be attached to the patient soon after his admission to hospital. Care must be taken also to ensure that all concerned know what operation is proposed and, where an operation may be performed on either side of the body, such as ligation of varicose veins or herniorrhaphy, it is clearly understood which side is to be operated on. It is wise, therefore, to check with each patient immediately before the induction of anaesthesia which side has been causing him trouble.

5

Pre-operative investigation of patients with disease of the heart and lungs

Students and residents know intuitively that the anaesthetist is especially concerned about the pre-operative condition of the heart and lungs, yet few understand exactly why. In this chapter, the principles underlying pre-operative cardiopulmonary assessment, in patients in whom disease is suspected, will be considered.

THE PATIENT WITH HEART DISEASE

Most patients with heart disease withstand the pharmacological and physiological stresses of general anaesthesia successfully. Nevertheless, the diseased heart is at risk during anaesthesia and in the post-operative period, for a number of important reasons.

Arrhythmia. The patient with an ischaemic myocardium may exhibit abnormal patterns of electrical conduction in the heart muscle which may be aggravated during anaesthesia, either because of a direct effect of the drugs used or as a consequence of inadvertent hypoxia.

Myocardial failure. The failing heart has a reduced ability to compensate for abnormal stresses or hypoxia during or after surgery, adjustments to blood loss and transfusion, and the circulatory disturbances associated with the institution of intermittent positive pressure ventilation.

Previous infarction. Anaesthesia and operation enhance the risk of another infarct, surgery occurring during the acute stages of recovery from myocardial infarction (the first three weeks) being associated with a mortality in excess of 50 per cent. A recent myocardial infarction is an indication for postponement of surgery which is not urgent, ideally for a period not less than 12 months.

Important points in pre-operative assessment
History. The patterns of previous illness should be noted with special reference to the frequency of attacks of cardiac failure, the

occurrence of, and precipitating factors in, chest pain, the need for admission to hospital and drug therapy. The capacity for exercise should be noted; a patient who gives a history of previous myocardial infarction but who has been free of symptoms for the past year presents less risk than the patient who suffers recurring attacks of angina at rest, and for which drug treatment is required, even although there has been no acute episode of infarction.

A history suggestive of myocardial failure such as swelling of the abdomen or ankles or attacks of dyspnoea should be noted. In the patient with stenosis of the mitral valve, a recent history of haemoptysis would suggest that the cardiac function may be difficult to control.

The routine clinical examination is important in confirming the impressions obtained from the history. It is essential to obtain a straight X-ray of the chest which will provide information about the size of the heart and its outline appearance, and may also indicate the presence of established pulmonary oedema.

The electrocardiogram should be obtained in all such patients; indeed there is a strong case for undertaking this type of investigation in all patients who are more than 40 years of age irrespective of the presence of symptoms and signs. The ECG should be examined for abnormal rhythm, evidence of ventricular enlargement, ischaemia, and infarction if present. It should be remembered that patients who have in fact suffered myocardial infarction may present in the surgical departments of the hospital with symptoms and signs which suggest surgical emergency, notably peritonitis.

The concentration of electrolytes in the serum of patients with heart disease should be measured before operation. In particular, it should be remembered that treatment with diuretics may cause abnormal losses of potassium; the blood urea concentration may be an important clue to renal impairment in patients with established cardiac failure.

If there is associated or co-existing pulmonary disease, it is important to measure the arterial oxygen tension (Pa_{O_2}) and the haemoglobin concentration should be known also.

THE PATIENT WITH PULMONARY DISEASE

The significance of pulmonary disease in a patient awaiting anaesthesia and operation is not connected with the fact that the anaesthetist may use the lungs as a route of administration of drugs; although the uptake of the inhalation anaesthetics may be impaired, for example in the patient with chronic bronchitis, this problem is not insuperable. The real difficulty relates to the *reserves* of lung function and whether or not these will be sufficient to allow the patient to withstand the physiological impairment, which is a consequence of the operation, so that adequate lung function can be ensured in the post-operative period. The following considerations apply:

— Where neuromuscular blocking drugs have been used, there is inevitably a small impairment of ventilatory capacity for several hours after operation. A patient with diminished ventilatory capacity, as a result of disease, may be at risk from developing post-operative ventilatory failure if the danger is not recognised and appropriate monitoring is not instituted.

— We have explained on page 23 that there is an increase in right-to-left shunting of blood within the lungs as a consequence of anaesthesia and the effects of abdominal surgery may aggravate this effect. For example, the patient who has undergone upper abdominal surgery can be expected to have a reduction of the arterial PO_2 of 3 to 4 kPa in the post-operative period (breathing air). This reduction will continue for 2 to 3 days after operation. This effect is a consequence of the anaesthetic initially, but wound pain, pneumoperitoneum and distension of bowel are the principal factors beyond the first 2 hours after surgery. These surgical factors may diminish the ventilatory capacity also.

— Excessive production of secretions by the bronchial mucosa may cause additional respiratory embarrassment to the patient who is unable to expectorate as a consequence of pain or debility, or both. Retained secretions will lead eventually to absorption collapse of segments of the lung.

Pre-operative assessment

Most of the important clues are to be found in the history. Questioning should be directed to the frequency and extent of previous illness related to the lungs, with special reference to the need for antibiotic therapy and admission to hospital. The occurrence of breathlessness is an estimate of the patient's tolerance of exercise and should be noted. The quantity of sputum production and the quality and colour of the expectorate are important, as is the patient's smoking habit. Even in the absence of a history of pulmonary disease, the heavy smoker can be expected to have an abnormally high sputum production.

The clinical examination of the chest will reveal signs of localised lung disease, and the general signs of chronic bronchitis and emphysema in the more severe cases, but it is worth remembering that a patient with seriously limited lung function may exhibit few abnormal signs on percussion and auscultation of the chest and that the important pointers are to be found in the history. The presence of finger clubbing is a valuable sign of intrapulmonary sepsis. Special attention should be paid to the configuration of the chest, for example the presence of marked kyphoscoliosis is almost invariably associated with diminished ventilatory function and chronic inflammatory changes in the lung tissue.

The chest should be X-rayed and special attention should be paid to the configuration of the chest wall in advanced disease; evidence of fibrosis and emphysema of the lung fields may be obvious but often abnormal changes, if any, are non-specific.

As a general rule, all patients undergoing abdominal surgery, with or without symptoms referable to the lungs, and all patients with a history of pulmonary disease should be X-rayed before anaesthesia and operation. Apart from a possible role in evaluation, the pre-operative chest X-ray provides a baseline in the event of respiratory problems in the post-operative period.

Lung function tests

Arterial blood should be sampled for the estimation of Po_2, Pco_2 and pH. Where there is pre-existing hypoxaemia (Po_2 less than 8 kPa, breathing air), and the patient is about to undergo abdominal surgery, it is unlikely that adequate oxygenation can be maintained in the post-operative period without artificial ventilation for 1 to 2 days and oxygen enrichment of the inspired gas.

If there is carbon dioxide retention (Pco_2 more than 6 kPa) before operation, it should be appreciated that the patient is likely to be dependent on the 'hypoxic drive' to ventilation and that excessive enrichment of the inspired oxygen concentration during spontaneous breathing may, paradoxically, aggravate ventilatory depression. In such patients, it may be desirable to institute positive pressure ventilation both during the operation and, if necessary, in the post-operative period.

Although there is a wide range of spirometric tests, few of these are of much value in pre-operative assessment. One exception is the measurement of the vital capacity and the forced vital capacity (FVC) (Fig. 5.1). In the former, the patient exhales to a spirometer at a rate of his choice until no more gas can be expelled from the lungs. The forced vital capacity is the same manœuvre undertaken

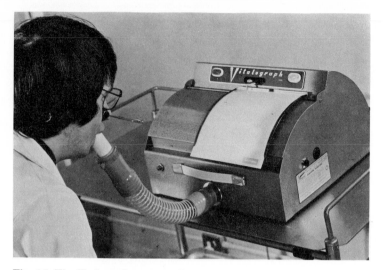

Fig. 5.1 The Vitalograph apparatus in use.

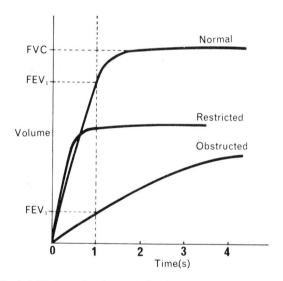

Fig. 5.2 Typical Vitalograph spirograms for three conditions. (1) Normal. (2) Restricted: patient with fibrosed lungs or limited chest movement as a result of obesity, rib cage disease, pain of an abdominal wound or loss of lung tissue (following pneumonectomy for example). (3) Obstructed: patient with airways narrowing such as asthma. Note that only in the obstructed condition is there a delay in the ability to expel gas from the lungs rapidly. Thus, FEV_1 as a proportion of FVC is a useful index of airways narrowing.

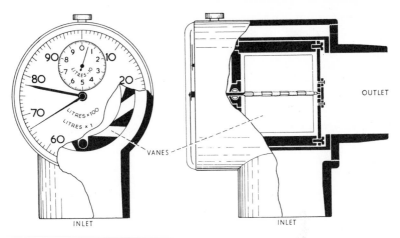

Fig. 5.3A This diagram shows the working principle of the Wright respirometer. Gases passing via the inlet, drive the vanes and the flow is recorded on the dials.

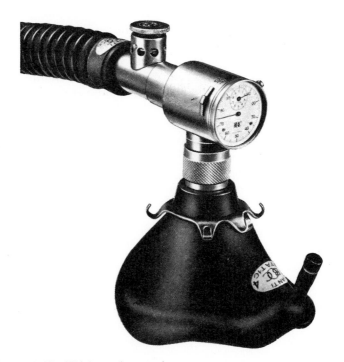

Fig. 5.3B The Wright respirometer in use.

in the minimum period of time. In the case of an adult of average size, the vital capacity should be in the range 3 to 5.5 litres. The effect of upper abdominal surgery will reduce this by about 55 per cent in the first 2 days after operation. The patient with restrictive lung disease will suffer the same percentage impairment so that if the pre-operative vital capacity is only 900 ml, he must undertake a maximum ventilatory effort to achieve a tidal volume of 400 to 450 ml. Not only would this be exhausting for the patient, but any further reduction in the tidal volume would lead inevitably to ventilatory failure.

The fraction of the forced vital capacity expired in 1 second (FEV_1) expressed as a percentage of FVC is a useful index of the airways resistance (Fig. 5.2). A normal subject should be able to achieve greater than 75 per cent, while a value less than 50 per cent denotes severe airways narrowing which may be associated with ventilatory failure in the post-operative period because of an unacceptably high work load of breathing.

In addition to the foregoing assessments, it may be of value to obtain bacteriological culture of a specimen of sputum together with an indication of the sensitivity of pathogens to antibiotics. Although it is established that there is little merit in the routine use of prophylactic antibiotic therapy in the patient who is undergoing surgery, there may be considerable advantage in delaying operation for 5 to 7 days to allow the physiotherapist to institute breathing exercises to promote the expectoration of sputum, and to enable antibiotic therapy to reduce the amount of bacterial contamination.

The Wright respirometer may be used to measure vital capacity and is particularly valuable for assessing the adequacy of the tidal volume after anaesthesia (Fig. 5.3).

6

Intravenous therapy

The ability to set up an intravenous infusion quickly and confidently under any circumstances is a great asset in any doctor and is essential to the anaesthetist, who may have to do so under very difficult conditions. Provided there is no contra-indication and adequate assistance is available during anaesthesia, it is often easier to set up an infusion after anaesthesia has been induced as the veins dilate and the procedure is not painful to the patient.

THE CHOICE OF INFUSION FLUID

For short-term management during anaesthesia and for the first 2 days of the post-operative period, it is important to remember that the patient who is deprived of oral intake has an average daily need of about 2.5 litres of water, 140 mmol of sodium and 100 mmol of chloride in each 24 hours. Assuming that the patient is in a satisfactory state of fluid and electrolyte balance before operation, other ion losses such as potassium and calcium can be ignored. Water losses may be increased substantially in a warm environment or where there are prolonged losses from the lungs as a result of the inhalation of dry gas during anaesthesia, or from serous surfaces during long operative procedures.

These simple guidelines would not be adequate for the management of the patient who is incapable of a normal oral intake for periods extending beyond 48 hours or for those who may suffer abnormal losses of water and electrolytes, for example from fistulae. For such patients, and indeed for all patients who are undergoing parenteral fluid therapy, a carefully maintained fluid and electrolyte balance chart is the basis of good management.

The choice of infusion fluid depends on the indications for the infusion.

Glucose and distilled water
Dextrose injection BP 5 per cent W/V contains 50 grams of anhydrous dextrose per litre of water. Although the solution contains

190 calories per litre, it is of little value as a source of nutrition in the surgical patient, and is used as a means of infusing the requirement of water, without electrolyte, as an isotonic solution.

Sodium chloride injection BP 0.9 per cent W/V

This solution, sometimes referred to as 'normal saline', contains 150 mmol of both sodium and chloride per litre.

It will be appreciated that the daily requirements of water, sodium and chloride are more than adequately met by the traditional post-operative regimen for an average adult of 1.5 to 2 litre of 5 per cent dextrose in water and 1 litre of normal saline, although it is worth noting that the chloride content is greater than necessary.

Compound sodium lactate injection BP (Hartmann's solution: Ringer–Lactate solution)

This solution, sometimes called 'balanced salt solution', contains 131 mmol of sodium, 5 mmol of potassium, 2 mmol of calcium, 111 mmol of chloride and 29 mmol of bicarbonate (as lactate). The solution is designed to be almost identical in composition to the patient's extracellular fluid. It follows, therefore, that this would be a more suitable solution to use for routine maintenance therapy in place of normal saline but the almost universal preference for the latter is traditional and, in practice, there is no serious objection to this. Hartmann's solution is preferred by most anaesthetists as a 'background infusion' during anaesthesia itself for procedures which are expected to last longer than 30 minutes. Provided renal function is normal, the recommended practice is to give 1 litre of Hartmann's solution in the first hour of anaesthesia and 500 ml per hour thereafter, in addition to measurable fluid losses which should be replaced with the whole blood or another plasma expander as appropriate.

During anaesthesia, several hormonal changes occur which have important implications for fluid and electrolyte balance. There is substantial and inappropriate secretion of anti-diuretic hormone (ADH) while the adrenal cortex increases its production of aldosterone. ADH inhibits renal secretion of free water (water unaccompanied by ions in isotonic concentration) whereas aldosterone promotes the retention of sodium. Because of these factors, water as 5 per cent dextrose solution and normal saline should not be given in amounts which exceed the anticipated losses. In the presence of satisfactory renal function, however, Hartmann's solution is capable of maintaining the composition and volume of the extracellular fluid while excesses can still be excreted by the kidney.

In the presence of renal disease, and in patients with myocardial failure, parenteral fluid therapy must be approached with caution. In broad terms, it can be said that the administration of fluids can be restricted to the anticipated losses only, and even then careful monitoring of the cardiovascular responses to fluid infusion is essential.

Blood

Normally blood is transfused when blood has been lost. It may be given before operations to correct anaemia. In this case, concentrated cells are often used but whole blood may be infused slowly where concentrated cells are not readily available. To counteract acute haemorrhage, however, whole blood, correctly grouped and cross-matched, is used. On occasion, a proportion of the measured blood loss may be replaced by the use of Hartmann's solution, or a suitable blood volume expander such as plasma, dextran, etc. (see below). When an anaesthetist commences the administration of blood during anaesthesia, he must ensure that the bottles of blood being transfused are those which have been previously grouped and cross-matched for the patient. Careful checking of the name and group on the bottle with those on the patient's case sheet is essential to avoid accidents. This is particularly important during anaesthesia when transfusion reactions are more difficult to recognise. Unexplained tachycardia, hypotension and oozing at the operation site may indicate the use of the wrong blood. The late consequences of a mis-matched transfusion are renal failure and jaundice as a result of haemolysis. It is important also to remember that the potassium concentration in the serum of the stored blood may be much greater than that of the patient's serum and that the pH is low.

Blood stored in a refrigerator will be transfused at a temperature below that of the body, the difference varying with the time lapse between removal and transfusion, and the rate of transfusion. With slow transfusions of relatively small amounts of blood, the low temperature of the blood is of little consequence. When large quantities of cold blood are transfused rapidly, however, a severe reduction in body temperature may result leading to cardiac arrest. Steps must be taken, therefore, to warm the blood to body temperature. This may be done by warming the bottle or container, or by passing the blood through a coil immersed in warm water (Fig. 6.1).

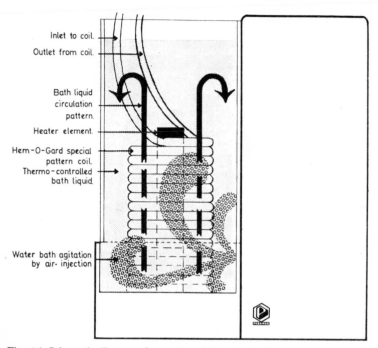

Inlet to coil.
Outlet from coil.
Bath liquid circulation pattern.
Heater element.
Hem-O-Gard special pattern coil.
Thermo-controlled bath liquid.
Water bath agitation by air-injection

Fig. 6.1 Schematic diagram of operation of Hem-0 Gard blood warming equipment.

In the transfusion of blood for the treatment of anaemia, it should be remembered that the elderly and those with a predisposition to cardiac failure may be placed at risk from excessive expansion of the circulating blood volume. Thus, slow infusion with careful monitoring of the patient is essential. The traditional acid–citrate–dextrose additive to whole blood reduces the stores of 2,3-diphosphoglycerate (2–3 DPG) with consequent impairment of the oxygen carriage of the transfused blood. Thus, paradoxically, the circulation may be embarrassed with no net improvement in the oxygen carriage as a result of treatment. Increasingly, citrate–phosphate–dextrose is being employed as a preservative and this has a less deleterious effect on 2–3 DPG.

Plasma
The need for plasma proteins, as opposed to whole blood, arises in two circumstances. Reconstituted dried plasma obtained from small donor pools may be transfused while blood is being obtained and cross-matched. This will restore the circulating volume but

will not replace the oxygen-carrying capacity of the blood which has been lost. In patients who are hypovolaemic and in electrolyte imbalance, plasma may be used to expand the circulatory volume and ensure adequate renal perfusion before administering aqueous electrolyte solutions. Even when plasma has been obtained from small groups of donors, there remains the risk of transmitting serum hepatitis. The manifestations of this may vary from a minor upset in liver function to severe jaundice and may prejudice the life of a seriously ill patient. For this reason, among others, plasma substitutes have been developed. Where the need is less urgent but it is desired to give a protein-containing solution, albumin (plasma protein solution) has replaced the use of whole plasma, as the hazards of hepatitis and other reactions are associated with the globulin fraction in the plasma. Other preparations such as concentrated platelets for use in platelet deficiency or cryoprecipitate for use in haemophiliacs are also available.

Plasma substitutes

A plasma substitute such as dextran (Dextran, Dextraven, Macrodex) may be given if blood or plasma are not readily available. This is a sugar solution containing large molecules (average molecular weight 70 000) with a high osmotic pressure which acts as a plasma expander. A reduction in post-operative phlebothrombosis is also claimed where Dextran 70 has been given during and after operation. Rheomacrodex is a solution of smaller molecular weight (average—40 000). Although it has a short half-life of about 3 hours in the body, it will restore the blood volume and may increase renal output by reducing the viscosity of blood after a considerable amount of blood has been given. However, excessive quantities result in the production of a highly viscid urine. 'Haemaccel' is a fractionated gelatin compound which, in addition to Dextran 70, is enjoying current popularity as a synthetic plasma expander.

Sodium bicarbonate solution

This is usually available as a concentration of 1 mol/ml and is given for the correction of metabolic acidosis. In most circumstances, the extent of metabolic acidosis should be determined accurately by deriving the base deficit. However, in emergencies when massive transfusion has been necessary, the infusion of not more than 100 mmol of sodium bicarbonate should be given without waiting for the laboratory data.

Intravenous feeding

In some patients, it is necessary to provide not only fluid but calorie requirements by the intravenous route for a considerable period. Special fluids are available which allow adequate calories to be given in relatively low fluid volumes. Preparations of amino-acids for intravenous use are available also (see p. 156).

APPARATUS AND TECHNIQUE

The choice or apparatus with which to set up the infusion is of importance. The container of the infusion fluid may be a glass bottle or a disposable plastic pack. The choice of administration set will depend on what is supplied in each hospital. There is a wide range of needles and cannulae available for use with the administration set.

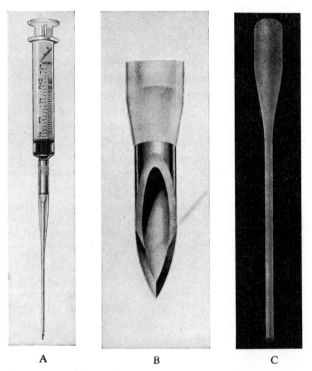

A   B   C

Fig. 6.2 The Medicut cannula. (A) shows the syringe, needle and cannula assembled for venepuncture. (B) shows the tapered cannula closely fitting the needle. (C) shows the blunt cannula which remains in the vein when the needle and syringe are withdrawn. Long polypropylene cannulae are available for use in conjunction with this set. When inserted through C they may be used to deliver irritant solutions into large veins or to measure the central venous pressure.

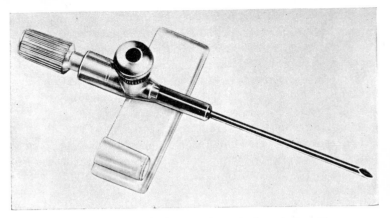

Fig. 6.3 The Viggo needle. Injections may be made through the rubber diaphragm on the top of the needle. The plastic plug in the hub of the needle may be removed and injections or infusions delivered by this route.

Although a needle may be inserted into the vein, there is a high probability that it will be extruded to the tissues. For this reason, it is preferable to use some form of cannula.

A typical cannula is illustrated in Figure 6.2. There is an inner metal needle and an outer plastic cannula. The combined unit is inserted into the vein and the needle is withdrawn, leaving the blunt cannula free in the vein. These cannulae, though most frequently used for intravenous infusions, may be used for repeated injections or sampling from within a vessel. In this case, a sterile rubber-capped plug is inserted into the end of the cannula. For repeated intravenous injections, special needles such as those shown in Figures 6.3 and 6.4 may be used.

In infants, a finer needle with a polythene tube extension similar to that in Figure 6.4 may be inserted in a convenient scalp vein.

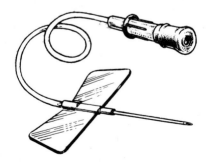

Fig. 6.4 The Abbott Butterfly needle. Injections given through the rubber diaphragm attached to the needle by a plastic tube.

Longer polythene cannulae may be used for prolonged continued infusion. These may be inserted through a short polythene cannula although there are several purpose-designed sets for 'no-touch' insertion of such cannulae (see Chapter 19).

A tapered polythene cannula may be introduced by direct exposure of the vein. It should be of wide bore and may be used for fast running infusions.

Usually, the anaesthetist requires an infusion which will allow a rapid controllable flow for a relatively short period—perhaps 24 hours. For this purpose, the short plastic cannulae are ideal. When

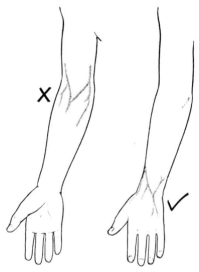

Fig. 6.5 Possible sites for setting up infusions. If the veins round the wrist and the back of the hand are chosen, greater mobility of the limb is possible without dislodging the needle or cannula.

an infusion is expected to run for several days and speed is not essential, the long thin polythene cannula is more suitable. The long, narrow-bore tubing offers considerable resistance to the flow of fluid into the vein and thus infusion takes place at a slower rate. When electrolytes are being replaced or when more irritant solutions are being delivered into larger, free running veins, these considerations are not important. Nutrient infusions, however, being more viscous, should be administered through the wide tapering cannula.

The site chosen for the venepuncture is of considerable importance (Fig. 6.5). The veins of the antecubital fossa, although very tempting and usually of considerable size, are less suitable for infusion during an operation. Movement of the elbow tends to displace the point or impede the flow through the cannula, and other sites are preferred. Among these are the veins available at the wrist and on the back of the hand. An infusion inserted here is readily accessible to the anaesthetist during the operation and injections can be made into it without disturbing the surgical procedure. The wrist can be splinted easily, if necessary, although often this is undesirable, and after operation the patient should be allowed full movement of the hand, provided care is taken to secure the cannula at the point at which it enters the skin. Normally in a right-handed person it is preferable to set up an infusion in the left hand. This point is often overlooked.

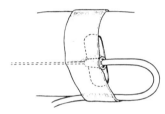

Fig. 6.6 If the apparatus is secured in the manner shown, traction on the tubing is less likely to dislodge the cannula.

As a rule, the leg should not be used for infusions as this may cause phlebitis, particularly if irritant solutions are used or if the infusion has been in existence for more than 48 hours. As the venous blood flow in the leg is less rapid than in the arms, and the leg veins are of larger size, leg vein thrombosis is more likely to occur and may be followed by serious consequences such as pulmonary embolism.

Before setting up an intravenous infusion, the doctor should ensure that everything, from the bottle of infusion fluid to the swabs and tape to secure the cannula, is immediately to hand. It is wise to secure a loop of the giving set at the site of connection to the cannula to prevent traction on the cannula (Fig. 6.6).

Transfusion under pressure
Under certain circumstances, it may be desirable to administer fluids, particularly blood, under pressure. Two methods are shown. A second chamber of the giving set containing a ball valve may be compressed to force the fluid into the patient (Fig. 6.7). This method should be employed if the fluid is in a rigid container.

Alternatively, a compressible cuff may be placed round an infusion bag (Fig. 6.8). The bulb is used to inflate the cuff to a pressure which is displayed on the gauge.

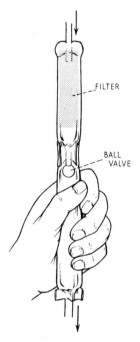

Fig. 6.7 A pressure transfusion set. The lower chamber is allowed to fill with blood and when the full chamber is again compressed the ball occludes the upper outlet and blood is forced down the tubing to the patient.

When it is desired to infuse fluid into a child with fine veins, or to give a drug in carefully metred doses to any patient, a specially designed infusion pump such as the IVAC may be employed.

Blood filters

Although the standard infusion apparatus for blood incorporates a fine mesh which acts as a filter for aggregates which may have formed during the storage period, there is evidence that small aggregates can pass through these filters. Some authorities believe that these particles may form small emboli, notably in the lungs, and suggest that this may cause or contribute to the 'shock lung' syndrome. Accordingly, if more than 1 litre of blood is to be administered a micropore filter (Fig. 6.9) should be incorporated in the infusion system.

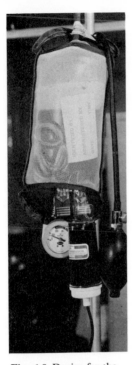

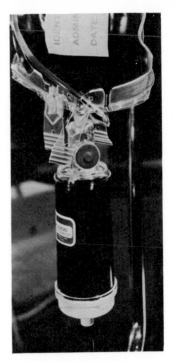

Fig. 6.8 Device for the
administration of blood to
a vein under pressure.
The bag containing blood
is enclosed in a cuff which
is inflated by squeezing
the bulb. The pressure
gauge is designed to show
the maximum safe
pressure which can be
used.

Fig. 6.9 Blood filter.

BLOOD LOSS ESTIMATIONS

Often it is not clear when to begin blood replacement and when
to discontinue it. Ideally, of course, blood volume should be
measured and haematocrit readings may be useful also. Often,
however, such measurements are impracticable and the value of
haemoglobin or haematocrit measurements will depend to a large
extent on the degree of haemo-concentration or haemo-dilution.
Thus it is important to consider the clinical indications for transfusion and the indications that transfusion has been adequate (Fig.
6.10).

By weighing the swabs which have been used during operation and comparing them with dry swabs it is possible to calculate the amount of blood which has been lost. It is also possible to wash the blood from the swabs and, by using a colorimeter, to measure the quantity lost.

When blood is lost, the peripheral circulation is reduced and the blood flow through the extremities, as measured by the plethysmograph, decreases. Only when this process can no longer compensate for the haemorrhage does the heart rate increase. When

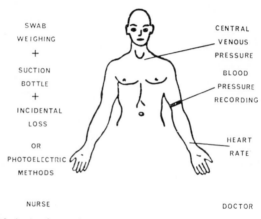

Fig. 6.10 Methods of assessing blood loss. The methods in which the nurse assists are shown on the left of the diagram.

the increase is no longer adequate to compensate for the blood loss, the arterial pressure decreases. This is shown in Fig. 6.11.

When blood loss is overt and appears likely to continue, it is desirable that replacement should be commenced before the onset of tachycardia and certainly before the arterial pressure has decreased markedly. Similarly, provided other causes of tachycardia and hypotension can be excluded, it is desirable to continue the transfusion until the arterial pressure and the pulse rate have returned to normal. Some indication of the adequacy of blood replacement can be gained by observing the filling of the neck veins when the patient is lying flat or with the head slightly raised. The central venous pressure may be measured more accurately by means of a cannula passed into the superior or inferior vena cava and attached to a saline manometer. A stable central venous pressure is another indication that replacement of blood loss has been adequate (see p. 170).

Blood volume and haematocrit measurements on the day following operating will indicate whether the blood volume and haemoglobin concentration have been restored to normal. Blood volume measurements, using either a dye dilution technique or dilution method with radioactive isotopes, can be performed in theatre and during major operations the blood volume is regularly monitored in this way.

HAEMORRHAGE AND TRANSFUSION

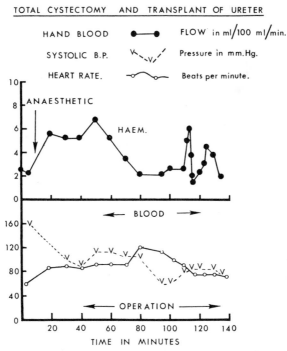

Fig. 6.11 The effects of haemorrhage and transfusion on blood flow, blood pressure and heart rate during surgery.

It is not possible in this chapter to deal extensively with all the problems associated with intravenous therapy. Remember when setting up an infusion to consider what you are trying to replace and the most logical method of replacing it. Never give blood if it is not indicated but do not hesitate to use blood where it is indicated, bearing in mind the replacement of blood volume and of haemoglobin with its oxygen-carrying capacity. Where possible, measure the blood loss. Blood volume measurements are an obvious guide to the amount of blood substitute to be administered and the haematocrit will give some indication of the haemoglobin concentration. Knowledge of the electrolyte values in the blood will allow the correct amount and type of electrolyte to be replaced. In the same way, acid–base measurements allow acidosis or alkalosis to be corrected.

In transfusing small children, note that their blood volume is approximately 110 ml per kg of body weight and that 500 ml of blood to a small child may represent a considerable proportion of the normal blood volume. Try neither to under-transfuse nor to over-transfuse. On the one hand, the heart has to beat faster to compensate for the deficiency in blood volume; on the other hand, the administration of excessive quantities of blood will impose a strain on the heart.

The control of intravenous infusions in general is a matter requiring co-operation between surgeon, anaesthetist and biochemist. Remember that if the need for large quantities of blood is anticipated, the blood bank must be warned in plenty of time as there may be difficulty in providing your requirements at a moment's notice.

7

The administration of a general anaesthetic

An anaesthetic can be divided into two phases: *induction* and *maintenance*. These may merge imperceptibly or there may be a fairly obvious demarcation between them. Induction of anaesthesia is considered to last from the moment when the anaesthetic is commenced until the requisite level of anaesthesia has been achieved for whatever operation is contemplated. This may take a few minutes or a considerable time, depending upon the method chosen and on the skill of the anaesthetist.

INDUCTION OF ANAESTHESIA

This is usually achieved by intravenous injection of suitable agents or by inhalation of gaseous anaesthetics, or vapours of volatile anaesthetic liquids. Before selecting a method, several questions must be answered:

— What is the safest method of induction?
— What is most pleasant for the patient?
— Which is the easiest and most practicable method under the circumstances?

The safety of each method lies in the avoidance of the complications associated with induction. These are regurgitation as the oesophageal sphincter relaxes, hypoxaemia (associated with coughing, bucking or laryngeal spasm), respiratory depression, and a decrease in arterial pressure resulting in circulatory insufficiency. For example, the inhalation of diethylether avoids the risk of sudden respiratory or cardiovascular depression, although the relative risk of coughing, etc. is greater. A rapid induction with i.v. thiopentone followed by suxamethonium may hasten the conditions for tracheal intubation, thus minimising the risks of regurgitation, although respiratory and cardiovascular depression are more likely. Paradoxically the rapid induction techniques are still associated with a short period of risk of regurgitation at a time when the protective reflexes have been totally abolished. Thus there is no easy rule-of-thumb in the selection of the technique, and the experience of the anaesthetist and the general condition of the patient are important determinants of the choice.

Intravenous induction of anaesthesia

The drugs normally employed are described in Chapter 2. Here we describe only induction with thiopentone.

This drug should be made up in a 2.5 per cent solution in water. A suitable vein should be sought and exposed and the arm or wrist compressed proximally. Because of the risks of accidental injection

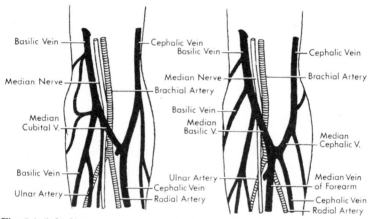

Fig. 7.1 (left) Showing arrangement of veins in region of cubital fossa (left arm). (right) Showing an alternative and frequently seen arrangement of veins in the same region (left arm).

to an artery (for example, thrombosis and gangrene may result), the vessel is palpated to ensure that it is not pulsating and the radial pulse also is checked to check that arterial pulsation has not been obliterated by the compression of the arm. A vein on the dorsum of the hand is commended as this is the site least likely to lead to accidental intra-arterial injection. If such a vein is not accessible, then one on the lateral aspect of the antecubital fossa should be selected. The use of the medial side of the antecubital fossa should be avoided whenever possible, because of the risk of injection into an artery; in addition the median nerve is vulnerable at this site (Fig. 7.1).

After these precautions have been observed, the needle is in-serted and blood aspirated to make sure that the needle is indeed in the vein. The colour of the aspirated blood will depend on several factors; in a well-sedated patient little oxygen is removed from the peripheral blood in the hand and, therefore, venous blood from the back of the hand may be bright red. There should be no signs of active pulsation of the blood into the syringe at any time, however. Pressure on the arm above the vein is now released and 1–2 ml of solution is injected. Thereafter, the injection is halted and a few moments are allowed for the drug to circulate. The patient is then asked whether he feels pain in the limb, at or below the point of injection. This is an essential precaution (p. 238).

If this test has been negative and the patient has not complained of pain, a further 2–3 ml should be injected, after which there should be a pause, and a further 2–3 ml of solution injected.

It is essential not to have fixed ideas as to the dose of thiopentone to be given before starting the injection. Small quantities should be injected at suitable intervals until the patient loses conscious-ness. If the patient is ill and has a slow circulation, longer pauses will be required between each 2–3 ml to allow the drug to circulate. The total dose of drug required to produce unconsciousness may vary widely, the ill, debilitated patient requiring perhaps 100 mg, the wrestler with a taste for alcohol requiring little less than 1 g. It is a popular practice to ask the patient to count, and when he ceases counting it is assumed that he has fallen asleep. However, some patients may continue counting in an automatic fashion beyond the point at which they can respond sensibly to questions asked in conversation. Many anaesthetists, therefore, prefer to speak to the patient and to note the point at which he ceases to answer or take part in the conversation.

When sleep has ensued, it is normally advisable to cease the injection of thiopentone as the drug is intended only to induce sleep and further administration may depress the myocardium. The induction is continued by administration of 70 per cent nitrous oxide in oxygen and, if necessary, a volatile agent such as halothane or ether may be added. If halothane is chosen, incre-ments of 0.5 per cent are added to reach perhaps 3–4 per cent depending on the response of the patient (see description of *over-pressure*, p. 6), but this concentration will be maintained only for a short time. If it is decided to use ether, which is more irritant, the addition of ether to the mixture will commence with a concen-tration of about 3 per cent and this is continued until no reaction to the vapour is obtained. Thereafter the concentration is increased slowly, allowing four breaths between each change of concentra-tion.

Inhalation induction of anaesthesia

This may be achieved in one of several ways. In the past, Inhalation anaesthesia was often induced with gaseous mixtures containing less than 20 per cent oxygen, sometimes none at all. This technique was used because it was considered to provide a rapid induction of anaesthesia which was pleasant for the patient and avoided some of the complications of the 'excitement stage' of Guedel's classification (p. 87). Not only did these techniques produce potentially dangerous hypoxia but inhalation of gaseous mixtures containing at least 20 per cent oxygen have been shown not to prolong the induction of anaesthesia significantly. Two techniques will be described.

In the first, the patient is asked to breathe a mixture of 70 per cent nitrous oxide in oxygen. This is continued until consciousness is lost as evidenced by loss of the eyelash reflex or the onset of a breathing pattern which is regular in rate or depth. A volatile agent, usually halothane, is now added in gradually increasing percentage, as described above, until the required level of anaesthesia is reached.

Bourne has described a technique in which a 6-litre reservoir bag is filled with a mixture containing 50 per cent each of cyclopropane and oxygen. The patient again breathes from a close-fitting mask and rebreathes into the bag; consciousness is lost after not more than 12 breaths. Anaesthesia may be continued with nitrous oxide and oxygen and a supplement. Alternatively, if the cyclopropane/oxygen mixture is inhaled for one minute, satisfactory operating conditions will persist for a further $1\frac{1}{2}$ minutes.

Pre-oxygenation

Where controlled ventilation with a mask may be difficult, in the obese patient for example, or dangerous, such as in the patient with a full stomach, a reserve of oxygen in the lungs is invaluable. If 100 per cent oxygen is breathed for 5 minutes, a large part of the nitrogen in the lungs will be washed out and replaced by oxygen. With this reserve in hand, the safe period of apnoea may be prolonged about fourfold in comparison with the patient who has breathed air only and tracheal intubation may be accompanied without hypoxia.

It is wise to practise the technique of pre-oxygenation for, although it is possibly unnecessary for many patients, it is always a valuable safeguard.

As we have now induced anaesthesia to a light level, administration of inhalation agents will continue until the anaesthesia is considered to be deep enough for the operation to be commenced. Obviously the criteria will vary with the particular operation and the degree of muscular relaxation required for its performance. No mention has been made, so far, of the use of muscle relaxants and these will be considered separately, as they involve the problems of assisted or controlled ventilation.

Before we can decide rationally when to reduce the concentration of volatile anaesthetics and judge that the patient is at a level of anaesthesia adequate for any particular operation, we must consider the signs of anaesthesia, as they will give a guide to the level of unconsciousness which has been or must be attained.

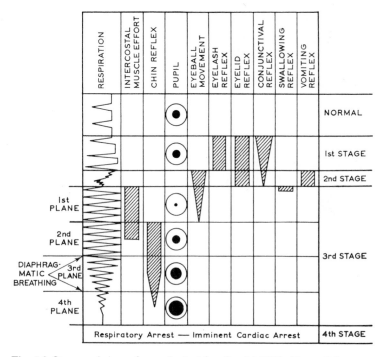

Fig. 7.2 Stages and signs of anaesthesia (after Geudel 1937). Many of these signs may be used to estimate the depth of unconsciousness resulting from other causes, e.g. head injuries.

THE SIGNS OF ANAESTHESIA

The stages and signs of anaesthesia, as described and taught normally, are those formulated by Guedel, and they apply to ether anaesthesia after premedication with atropine. A modified table of Guedel's signs is shown in Figure 7.2.

Many students are rather puzzled to see that the classical stages and signs about which they have read are not in evidence when modern anaesthetic techniques are used. There are, however, good reasons for this. We have discussed earlier (p. 8) the division of anaesthesia into its three parts—sleep, analgesia and muscular relaxation. It is this division of anaesthesia into its component parts and the use of specific drugs to produce them which has revolutionised anaesthesia. One may, for instance, produce apnoea, which does not occur until Stage IV in Guedel's classification, by the use of myoneural blockade without having produced either unconsciousness or indeed any analgesia. Similarly, it is possible, by rapid injection of a barbiturate, to produce apnoea although the patient will respond to a painful stimulus. It is for this reason that, using modern anaesthetic techniques, the anaesthetist must depend on other signs to identify the depth of anaesthesia.

Loss of consciousness

When thiopentone is used, it is not difficult to demonstrate that the patient has lost consciousness, for example he may be asked to count. Using inhalation methods, the distinction is not quite so clear but the onset of automatic (regular) breathing is a sure sign that consciousness has been lost. In addition, the loss of the eyelid reflex—the eyelash is stroked with the finger and the eyelid no longer closes—is a valuable guide to loss of consciousness. A further, but seldom used, test is to ask the patient to hold one arm in the air and when the arm falls to his side he is asleep.

When anaesthesia is continued with nitrous oxide and a volatile supplement in oxygen, the problem of inadvertent regaining of consciousness seldom arises. On rare occasions, patients in whom anaesthesia is maintained with nitrous oxide, oxygen and a muscle relaxant may complain that they remember incidents during an operation. This has occurred when no sedative premedication has been used, a limited dose of thiopentone has been given for induction, and anaesthesia has been maintained using nitrous oxide and more than 33 per cent of oxygen. In obstetric anaesthesia, the risk of depressing the baby has resulted in a tendency to reduce the dosage of narcotics and volatile anaesthetics and it is in this context that the problem of awareness occurs most frequently.

The use of hyoscine in premedication in place of atropine is believed by some to reduce this incidence of awareness during anaesthesia.

The routine use of a supplementary volatile agent with nitrous oxide and oxygen should abolish awareness in surgical practice but is associated with a slower recovery of consciousness.

The return of the eyelash reflex and movements of the eyelids and eyebrows in a patient who has received a myoneural blocking drug should suggest that the patient requires supplementation of the anaesthetic.

Assessment of analgesia (sensory blockade)

Here we are looking for the normal physiological reactions of the conscious person to pain, modified according to the degree of analgesia present and whether or not a muscle relaxant has been used.

Withdrawl from the painful stimulus. This may take the form of gross movement—a hand may be withdrawn from the surgeon's knife or the patient may draw up his knee. Such movement results when the level of anaesthesia is too light and a severe stimulus is applied. When the depth of anaesthesia is just insufficient for the operation to be performed and when a muscle relaxant has been used, the reaction may be restricted to slight movement of the fingers and hand or wrinkling of the forehead. The patient may move his head from side to side in a characteristic rocking fashion.

Phonation. Patients will normally cry out when hurt and, if it is possible during light-anaesthesia, some attempt at phonation is usually made. Obviously this is not possible when an endotracheal tube is in place.

Irregular breathing or breath-holding may be signs of inadequate analgesia for the operation being performed. Laryngeal stridor may be included under this heading.

A further group of signs are associated with *sympathetic overactivity*—part of the 'fight and flight' reaction; the skin is seen to be pale, cold and sweating, and the heart rate and the arterial pressure are increased.

Another important sign is *lachrymation*. These signs may be found at the beginning of the operation when the surgeon's skin incision is made, during operation if the anaesthetic becomes too light or in operations where intensely painful stimuli are inflicted at intervals. They are an indication to increase the depth of anaesthesia by increasing the concentration of the volatile agent. If only nitrous oxide and oxygen are administered in the gas mixture, the signs are an indication for the addition of a volatile agent to the mixture or for the administration of small doses of narcotics such as morphine 2–5 mg i.v.

Is muscular relaxation adequate?

The degree of muscular relaxation needed for any particular operation is a matter which can be decided by experience and a little foresight.

During diethylether anaesthesia, the anaesthetist may look for the signs in Guedel's classification to estimate the degree of muscular relaxation according to the *stage* of anaesthesia. Careful observation of these signs during inhalational anaesthesia will ensure that the appropriate level of anaesthesia is maintained throughout.

When minor procedures, such as the manipulation of a fracture, are to be carried out, it is possible, after anaesthesia has been induced, to test the relaxation in the limb concerned. It must be remembered, however, that, while a limb may be flaccid at rest, when painful manipulation is carried out the muscles may contract.

When myoneural blockade has been produced and ventilation is being controlled, it may be difficult for the anaesthetist to decide whether relaxation remains adequate. Although respiration may have been abolished by the original dose of muscle relaxant, in many cases the fact that respiration has not restarted is not of itself a sufficient indication that relaxation remains complete. While ventilation is controlled, the level of carbon dioxide in the blood may be reduced. This together with central depression by the anaesthetic drugs may account for continuing apnoea after the effect of the neuromuscular block has lessened. Some guides to the fact that relaxation has lessened are:

— *The surgeon may complain that the patient is 'tense'.* This is not always a reliable guide as surgeons tend to differ in their estimation of what is adequate relaxation. A particularly courteous surgeon may not wish to cause offence!
— If the anaesthetist observes the surgical wound in the abdomen, he may see that *bowel is being extruded* or that the peritoneum is retracted into the wound, or is tearing as it is being stitched.
— If ventilation is being controlled by manual compression of the reservoir bag, the anaesthetist may notice that the *pressure required to inflate the lungs to the same volume is increasing* and

that greater effort has to be used to inflate the lungs with the same volume of gas. If a mechanical ventilator is being used, it is possible that, to maintain the same tidal volume, a higher inflation pressure is required; if the ventilator is set to deliver a constant pressure, a reduced volume of gas may be delivered to the patient by the same pressure. These effects are a result of returning tone in the muscles of the chest wall and upper abdomen.

— If the anaesthetist does not appreciate these signs and compensates (for a reduced volume) by increasing the pressure in the reservoir bag, he may notice that the *arterial pressure is decreasing* without obvious reason. This is a result of the increased intrathoracic pressure reducing the venous return and, consequently, the cardiac output (see p. 166).

— There may be movement ('chewing') of the tracheal tube or the patient may make *spontaneous respiratory efforts*.

When muscular relaxation is seen to be inadequate in this way, the anaesthetic is either deepened, if inhalation agents only are being used, or, if muscle relaxants have been given, an appropriate supplementary dose of the relaxant agent is administered intravenously.

One must consider what signs are most likely to be shown by the patient under the circumstances of any given anaesthetic. If an opiate has been used in premedication and thiopentone has been given early in the anaesthetic, the patient's pupils are likely to be small throughout the anaesthetic in the absence of gross hypoxia or very severe painful stimuli. Similarly, when muscle relaxant drugs have been administered the eyeball will remain fixed while they are acting.

Provided the patient is adequately relaxed and hyperventilation is undertaken, some anaesthetists consider that the signs suggestive of inadequate analgesia are not of importance. However, this is precisely the situation in which a later complaint of awareness during surgery may occur. On the other hand, it has been shown that even under deep levels of anaesthesia where there are no outward signs that the patient is receiving painful stimuli, such stimuli in fact do reach the cerebral cortex and there is little indication that the patient is any the worse for this. The only method of blocking the passage of these impulses to the brain is by regional nerve block, that is blocking the impulses as they pass along nerves before they reach the spinal cord.

THE FURTHER MAINTENANCE AND CONCLUSION OF ANAESTHESIA

We have dealt at some length with the recognition of various signs during anaesthesia. If one understands what to look for and recognises the state in which the patient is during anaesthesia then appropriate action can be taken. Thus if the patient is inadequately anaesthetised, further increments of the intravenous analgesic or an increased concentration of the volatile agents can be given. If muscle relaxation is inadequate appropriate measures can be taken and if ventilation is inadequate this can be augmented. Similarly, by knowing the circumstances in which complications may occur, many can be prevented. By early recognition of the complications which do arise, prompt treatment will ensure anaesthesia continues smoothly.

We may, however, consider in further detail the administration of two types of anaesthetic.

Spontaneous respiration with inhalation agents

Anaesthesia may be induced either by intravenous or inhalation methods as mentioned in the section on induction of anaesthesia. The patient will have been anaesthetised to the level appropriate for the particular operation and the anaesthetist will watch for the signs which indicate that this level has been reached. He will then keep a regular check on the signs of anaesthesia at the level which he has chosen and, provided they are maintained, a low concentration of vapour such as 0.5 per cent to 1 per cent halothane will suffice for a prolonged period. Towards the end of operation, the level of anaesthesia may be lightened but the extent of this will depend on the depth to which anaesthesia has been carried and the nature of the operation. Thus if nitrous oxide, oxygen and halothane have been given, halothane may be discontinued as the wound is being closed. However, it is a matter of judgment and experience to ensure that the level of anaesthesia does not lighten excessively before the end of the surgical procedure. While it is desirable to have a patient regain consciousness within a few minutes of the termination of the operation, it is a risky procedure to try to maintain a very light level of anaesthesia, since it is at this level that vomiting, coughing and laryngeal spasm are most likely. Thus adequate anaesthesia should be maintained until one is in a position to deal with these complications during recovery from anaesthesia without interrupting the course of the operation.

Controlled ventilation using muscle relaxants

Anaesthesia will usually be induced by the use of an intravenous agent and a myoneural blocking drug will be given to paralyse the muscles. Thereafter a tracheal tube will be passed and ventilation controlled by manual or mechanical means. During the anaesthetic, the signs of inadequate analgesia and inadequate ventilation will be sought and the patient observed carefully to ensure that relaxation is adequate. Supplements of the analgesic or relaxant drugs will be given according to the indications, and these procedures will be continued throughout the operation. Once the peritoneum is closed, the patient, usually still apnoeic, will have to be prepared for the end of the operation and steps are now taken to restore spontaneous ventilation.

If the muscle relaxant is still considered to be acting, as shown by ease in closing the peritoneum, the appropriate antagonist is given. In the case of the non-depolarising drugs neostigmine in a dose of 2.5 to 5 mg intravenously is given. As this drug produces severe bradycardia, marked salivation and possibly bronchospasm, it is preceded by atropine, normally 1.2 mg administered intravenously. If spontaneous respiration does not follow the administration of these drugs, further steps may be necessary, in the light of the possible causes of continued apnoea. If hyperventilation has been performed throughout the operation, many anaesthetists will administer carbon dioxide 5–10 per cent for a limited number of breaths, say 10 to 20 ventilations. If tracheobronchial or pharyngeal suction is undertaken, the passage of the catheter into the trachea or into the pharynx is often sufficient, as a nonspecific stimulus, to cause spontaneous breathing. Where excessive depression by narcotic analgesics is suspected, antagonists such as nalorphine 1–2 mg or naloxone up to 0.4 mg may be given. As a rule, however, such drugs should not be necessary if the decisions about the dosage of narcotics during surgery have been appropriate.

When an endotracheal tube is in place, tracheobronchial suction, using a sterile catheter through the tube, may be employed to remove secretions.

As tracheobronchial suction may deplete the lungs' store of oxygen, it is essential to administer oxygen before and after suction to compensate for this. At this stage secretions should be cleared from the pharynx under direct vision using the laryngoscope. Thereafter, the tube is withdrawn from the trachea. Once the pharynx has been aspirated the same catheter should not be used again in the trachea, in case infection is introduced. At this stage,

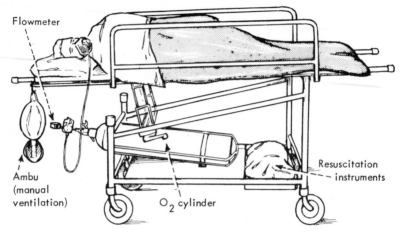

Fig. 7.3 Patient on tilting trolley awaiting transfer to the recovery room. The cylinder of oxygen lies below the trolley and the mechanism for tilting is above the cylinder.

the patient may be transferred to a tilting trolley and placed on her side (Fig. 7.3). Supplementary oxygen, up to 4 litres per minute by means of an Edinburgh mask, for example, should be given, particularly in patients with signs of cardiovascular or respiratory disease.

When the anaesthetist is satisfied that the patient is recovering and is fit to return to the ward, he should be handed over to the care of a responsible person. It is important to remember that, until this is done, the immediate responsibility for the patient's

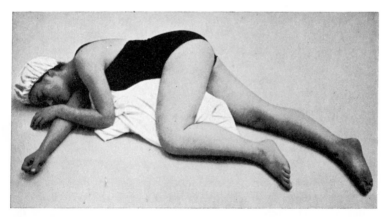

Fig. 7.4 The tonsillar position: the patient lies midway between the lateral and the prone positions, prevented from rolling face downwards by the pillow and the position of the arms and legs.

safety rests with the person who is giving the anaesthetic. A useful test at this stage, if muscle relaxant drugs have been given, is to ask the patient to put out the tongue or lift the head from the pillow. If this can be done, it is likely that the patient is in a safe state to return to the ward. When in doubt, the anaesthetist himself should see his patient safely back in bed, preferably in the tonsillar position (Fig. 7.4). In this position, the tongue falls forward, the airway remains clear and if vomiting or regurgitation should occur, the vomitus will flow away from the air passages (see p. 125). Never be rushed into starting another anaesthetic before you are satisfied with the condition of the previous patient. A few minutes' lack of supervision at this stage may undo hours of careful work in the theatre. It is also important to ensure that clear instructions for the patient's immediate post-operative care accompany him to the ward. These should be on the form used by the anaesthetist to record the drugs given in theatre, the heart rate and the arterial pressure. In this way, continuity of care in intravenous and analgesic therapy is improved.

8

Endotracheal intubation and endoscopy

The technique of laryngoscopy and intubation of the trachea is essential to the practice of anaesthesia. However, these simple skills are of value outside the operating theatre in a variety of circumstances, ranging from resuscitation of the new-born to the first aid management of the patient who has suffered cardiac arrest.

Indications for endotracheal intubation

Maintenance of a clear airway under difficult circumstances
If the anaesthetised patient is to lie on his side, on his face or in the head-down position, it may not be possible to maintain a clear airway using an oropharyngeal airway only. In obese subjects, particularly those who are edentulous, it may even be difficult to maintain the airway during anaesthesia even in the supine position. In all these circumstances, the insertion of a tracheal tube assures the airway.

Operations on the head, neck, mouth, throat and nose
In most of these procedures, the anaesthetist and the surgeon may be competing for access and the use of a face mask is impracticable; a tracheal tube and its connection is much less obtrusive.

Protection of the trachea
The presence of a cuffed tracheal tube prevents materials such as blood, mucus, pus or vomitus from gaining access to the trachea and the lungs. This is of particular importance for operations on the nose and mouth and in patients liable to vomit or regurgitate during anaesthesia, notably in obstetric practice and in patients with intestinal obstruction.

Reduction of respiratory dead space
The presence of a tracheal tube will reduce the physiological dead space by 30–40 per cent. This is of particular importance in the

small child in whom the use of a face mask might add to the respiratory dead space to such an extent as to cause ventilatory failure.

Facilitation of tracheobronchial toilet

A tracheal tube facilitates the passage of a suction catheter to the trachea and main bronchi for the aspiration of mucus and other undesired material. In the case of a discrete plug of mucus or more solid matter, bronchoscopy may be necessary. This procedure is described later in the present chapter. It should be noted here that a fibreoptic probe may be inserted through a tracheal tube for inspection of the bronchial tree and suction under direct vision. Once the tracheal tube is in position, fibreoptic endoscopy causes virtually no additional disturbance to the patient.

Controlled ventilation

In most circumstances in which it is intended to undertake artificial ventilation of the lungs by intermittent positive pressure means, the presence of a tracheal tube (except in patients in whom tracheostomy has been performed) is essential. However, these comments do not apply to the use of positive pressure ventilation for a few minutes in the resuscitation of the apnoeic patient. In these patients, the application of gas under pressure from a face mask (using an Ambu bag for example) is a first essential in treatment and satisfactory oxygenation of the arterial blood should be restored before tracheal intubation is attempted.

Therapeutic indications for endotracheal intubation

In the care of the unconscious, the absence of an adequate cough reflex warrants tracheal intubation to ensure protection of the airway from liquid material in the pharynx. In addition, the presence of the tube allows tracheobronchial toilet to be carried out at any time. Thus there are indications for endotracheal intubation in patients who have been severely poisoned by drugs such as barbiturates and in patients with head injury and cerebrovascular accidents.

In patients with post-operative respiratory insufficiency, the use of a tracheal tube may reduce the respiratory dead space sufficient to allow adequate ventilation until recovery of function (by the control of pain or the antagonism of myoneural blockade) has occurred.

In resuscitation of the new-born, the passage of a tracheal tube facilitates artificial ventilation and endotracheal suction. In other forms of resuscitation, such as the treatment, after the first few minutes, of cardiac arrest or drowning, the ability to pass a tracheal tube may be invaluable.

There are three essentials for the successful passage of a tube to the trachea:

1. Adequate relaxation of the muscles of the head, neck and larynx.
2. Satisfactory positioning of the head and neck.
3. The correct use of apparatus.

Anaesthesia for endotracheal intubation

Most commonly, the patient will have received an intravenous induction agent such as thiopentone which is followed immediately by the injection of a myoneural blocking drug such as suxamethonium. As soon as the myoneural block is established, the patient's lungs are ventilated with gas under pressure from a face piece and a reservoir bag and the patient is now ready for laryngoscopy and intubation. Alternatively, a deep level of anaesthesia may be induced with an inhalation anaesthetic such as halothane, ether or cyclopropane to the point at which the cough reflex is obtunded. In these circumstances, the conditions for laryngoscopy and intubation are obtained without the need for myoneural blockade.

The mouth, pharynx, laryngeal inlet and bronchial tree may be anaesthetised by the topical application of a local anaesthetic such as lignocaine 4 per cent. This technique is employed in situations in which the induction of general anaesthesia as a preliminary to tracheal intubation may be fraught with danger because of difficulties in maintaining the airway, such as in patients with fixed deformities of the cervical spine.

In the resuscitation room, it is common to find that the reasons demanding tracheal intubation are associated with unconsciousness so that the question of anaesthesia does not arise.

Posture of the patient

The neck should be slightly flexed and the head extended. This has been described as a position for 'sniffing the air'. It is illustrated correctly in Figure 8.1 from which it can be seen that the correct position results in a straight line from the mouth through the vocal cords to the trachea. The common mistake is to extend the neck and the head as shown in Figure 8.2 and the resulting difficulties are obvious. It is often the case that when the head

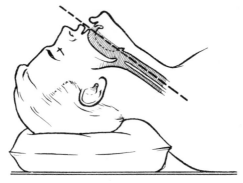

Fig. 8.1 The correct posture of head and neck for laryngoscopy. With the neck flexed and the head extended, the mouth, laryngoscope and trachea are in a straight line.

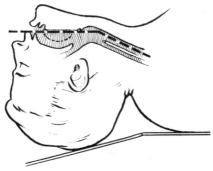

Fig. 8.2 The incorrect posture for laryngoscopy. With the neck extended and head extended, the trachea and laryngoscope blade are no longer in line.

is correctly positioned in a patient whose muscles are sufficiently relaxed to allow tracheal intubation, the mouth will open slightly, allowing entry to the blade of the laryngoscope. Thus, the need to use one's fingers to open the mouth is a sign that the positioning is incorrect.

Apparatus

The apparatus for direct or blind intubation of the trachea consists of laryngoscopes, tracheal tubes, aids to the introduction of the tracheal tube such as a malleable stilette, sprays for producing local analgesia of the larynx, and connectors to connect the tracheal tube to the anaesthetic apparatus or ventilator.

Laryngoscopes

Laryngoscopes may be divided into two groups, those with straight blades and those with curved blades. The first typified

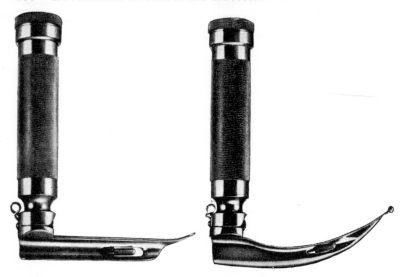

Fig. 8.3 The Magill laryngoscope.   **Fig. 8.4** The Macintosh laryngoscope.

by the Magill laryngoscope shown in Figure 8.3 is passed over the base of the tongue and the posterior surface of the epiglottis exposing the larynx in a straight line. As the posterior surface of the epiglottis is supplied by the vagus nerve, reflexes set up by the use of this instrument tend to cause laryngeal spasm and a deep level of general anaesthesia will be required to avoid this. The Macintosh laryngoscope (Fig. 8.4) was designed to pass over the base of the tongue but into the vallecula anterior to the epiglottis, an area which is supplied by the glossopharyngeal nerve. Figures 8.5 and 8.6 show the two instruments in use, and illustrate this point. The advent of the myoneural blocking drugs

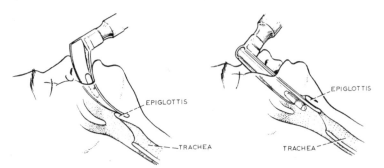

Fig. 8.5 The Macintosh laryngoscope in use. The blade tip is anterior to the epiglottis.

Fig. 8.6 The Magill laryngoscope in use. The blade tip is posterior to the epiglottis.

as an aid to laryngoscopy has lessened the need for the straight blade laryngoscope and the Macintosh blade is used most commonly in modern practice. However, the Magill blade continues to be of use in paediatric practice and in adults with deformities of the jaw or neck.

Endotracheal tubes
These vary considerably in design. The commonest example (Fig. 8.7) is a curved tube with an angled aperture for insertion to the trachea and a cuff which is fixed to the outer surface of the tube near its distal end. The cuff may be inflated with air to provide a seal between the outer part of the tube and the lining of the trachea. A small indicator balloon on the inflation catheter of the cuff serves to reassure the anaesthetist that the cuff is functioning adequately. Sometimes it is preferable to have a tube without a cuff;

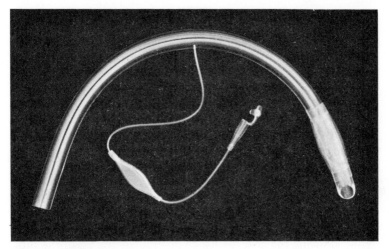

Fig. 8.7 A cuffed 'Portex' tube.

such 'plain' tubes may be used for insertion through the nose (nasotracheal intubation) or may be preferred in circumstances in which the trachea is particularly at risk from pressure, such as might result from inflation of a cuff.

In certain circumstances, such as operations in which the position of the head may be changed several times during surgery, for example neurosurgery, or in operations in which a gag is placed in the mouth and may obstruct the tracheal tube, such as in operations for the repair of a cleft palate or in tonsillectomy, reinforcement of the side of the tube may be required to prevent kinking or compression. Various forms of reinforced tubes are available. In some cases, a nylon spiral may be used to reinforce the wall of the tube, while an alternative is the use of a tapered tube, the narrow distal end being of a size suitable for insertion to the larynx, while the more proximal part (in relation to the anaesthetist) is constructed of thick plastic or rubber which is less compressible than is the more commonly used tube. In the past, the majority of the commonly used tracheal tubes were made of red rubber and were re-used many times. This had the disadvantage of the high cost and difficulty of sterilisation together with the risk of damage to the inflatable cuff when present. In many hospitals nowadays, tubes are made of plastic materials and are pre-packed and sterilised by the manufacturer with the intention that they be discarded after use.

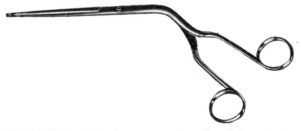

Fig. 8.8 The Magill intubating forceps, curved to allow their use in the mouth, are used to guide an endotracheal tube through the vocal cords.

Intubating forceps
(See Fig. 8.8.) This example designed by Magill is in common use. The instrument is of great value during nasotracheal intubation in allowing the anaesthetist to manipulate the tip of the tube to the laryngeal inlet. These forceps are also of value when it is necessary to insert a nasogastric tube after anaesthesia has been induced.

Laryngeal sprays
Laryngeal sprays have been designed to facilitate the deposition of a fine mist of local analgesic solution on the mucosa of the respiratory tract. This may be desirable even when general anaesthesia has been employed so that the reflexes caused by the tube as it passes into the trachea may be minimised. One such spray is shown in Figure 8.9.

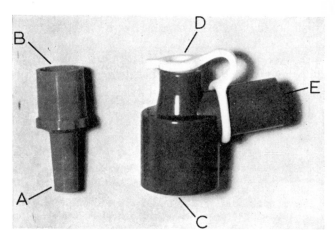

Fig. 8.9 The Portex endotracheal connector and swivel mount. This may be used as a unit by connecting A to the endotracheal tube, B to C and E to a catheter mount and thus to the anaesthetic machine. In this case, suction catheters may be passed into the trachea by lifting the cap D. Alternatively, using the modern British Standard connector, B may be joined directly to the delivery tube from the machine.

Connectors

The pre-packed plastic tubes have a plastic connector (for example Fig. 8.10) included in the package. Such a connector is simple in design and allows access for suction catheters easily. In earlier times, connectors were made of metal and were intended to be

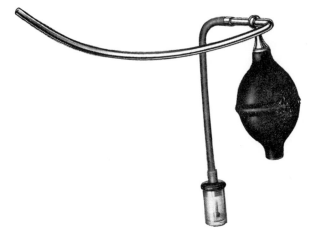

Fig. 8.10 The Forrester laryngeal spray. The container for the analgesic has a maximum capacity of 4 ml. The metal part of the spray fits the curvature of a Macintosh laryngoscope.

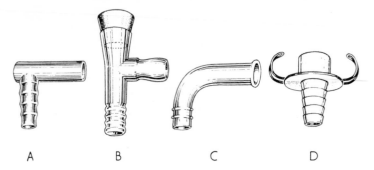

Fig. 8.11 Endotracheal tube connectors. A. The Rowbottom connector. The right angle causes turbulent flow which increases resistance during respiration. B. A suction connector. The rubber cork can be removed to allow the passage of a suction catheter without disconnecting the tube. C. A curved connector which reduces turbulence and thus the resistance to respiration. D. The Forrester connector. This connector is straight and of wide bore. Resistance to respiration is minimal and endotracheal suction is easily performed.

inserted to the proximal end of a rubber tracheal tube. These are illustrated in Figure 8.11 although they are rapidly becoming obsolete.

It is important to ensure that the endotracheal tube and its connector are of such diameter that the resistance to flow through them is not excessive. It is important to note that it is the narrowest part of the system that determines the magnitude of the resistance so that it is unwise to insert a connector to a tube unless it is of virtually the same diameter as the tube itself.

The technique of endotracheal intubation

Before commencing, it is important that everything should be at hand so that there is no delay once the procedure has started. The chosen laryngoscope should be tested to ensure that the light housed in the blade is working satisfactorily. It is particularly important to check that there is a suitable means of connecting the tracheal tube to the anaesthetic circuit or source of positive pressure ventilation. The internal diameter of the tube is given in millimetres on the outer wall and when the anaesthetist speaks of the 'size' of the tube it is this dimension that is referred to. The appropriate size of the tube is based on the patient's age. In the case of a child: the age in years should be divided by four and 4.5 is added to the answer. Thus a 6.5 mm tube would be appropriate for a child of 8 years. However, there are considerable variations in the size of the larynx and many anaesthetists may wish to have in addition a tube which is one size bigger and one size smaller than the predicted. For adult patients, the tube sizes ranging from 8.0 mm (for a small lady) to 10.0 mm (for a large man) should be employed.

A rough guide to the correct length of tube can be obtained by measuring the distance from the lobe of the ear to the angle of the mouth, for oral intubation, or the nose for nasal intubation. A tube cut to twice this length should reach from the incisor teeth or nostril to the mid-point to the trachea.

The laryngoscope is introduced into the patient's mouth along the right border of the tongue. The blade is slipped over the tongue until the epiglottis is visible. If a Magill laryngoscope is being

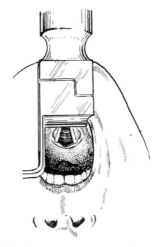

Fig. 8.12 The view of the larynx and trachea obtained on direct laryngoscopy.

used, the epiglottis is lifted forward, whereas if a Macintosh laryngoscope is used, the tip of the laryngoscope is inserted into the vallecula and the base of the tongue is lifted forward, carrying the epiglottis with it. A view such as shown in Figure 8.12 will be obtained. The novice is often tempted to lever the handle of the laryngoscope to a more vertical position. Not only does this endanger the teeth but it will tend to push the larynx upwards and away from the field of vision.

Assuming that a good view of the laryngeal inlet has been obtained and that there is no danger of the inhalation of vomitus or blood at the end of the operation, one may decide to spray the vocal cords and through the cords into the trachea with a local analgesic. A suitable spray is used and a total dose of not more than 4 ml of 4 per cent lignocaine is given. Similar qualifications apply to the use of local analgesic lubricants applied to the tube before insertion in the trachea. In patients who are undergoing surgery for the relief of intestinal obstruction, or operations on the mouth, throat or nose where blood may be present in the pharynx at the end of operation, a non-analgesic lubricant such as 'KY' jelly is preferred.

Where appropriate, the cuff of the tube is inflated with air at the same time as attempts are made to ventilate the lungs from a reservoir bag. The amount of air injected to the cuff should be just enough to prevent the audible return of the ventilating gas between the tube and the trachea.

Complications of endotracheal intubation

If there is difficulty in ventilating the patient's lungs, obstruction of the tube should be considered. The diagnosis can be confirmed by passing a finger into the mouth along the length of the tube. Kinking may be abolished by correct positioning of the head and sometimes the introduction of an oropharyngeal airway into the mouth will help to prevent kinking. Occasionally, an excessively long tube may have been passed into the right bronchus. As a check against this possibility, it is essential to ensure that both lungs can be inflated. If necessary, this should be checked by auscultation.

Sore throat is common following endotracheal anaesthesia and probably occurs in about 50 per cent of all patients at risk. The incidence may be reduced by care during the introduction of the tube and by the use of adequate lubrication. The use of gauze packs to absorb blood, during tonsillectomy for example, is an additional factor which predisposes to sore throat in the post-operative period. This minor but nevertheless annoying complication can be treated if necessary with mild analgesics and mouth washes.

Oedema of the larynx leads to laryngeal stridor and partial or complete obstruction of the airway. It is a rare complication of tracheal intubation in adults, but occurs more commonly in children. The treatment includes the inhalation of humidified oxygen or menthol vapour. In severe cases, helium–oxygen mixtures may be used and tracheostomy may be necessary if these more simple measures fail. Laryngeal granulomata and tracheal stenosis are serious complications of tracheal intubation, but are associated more commonly with prolonged intubation such as might be necessary in the intensive therapy unit.

SPECIAL TUBES AND BLOCKERS

We have considered endotracheal tubes which are normally passed to a point midway between the cords and the bifurcation of the trachea. However, more elaborate tubes are available for the special needs of thoracic surgery. Depending on the particular design, these may be passed into one or other main bronchus so that the anaesthetic may be maintained via one lung while the other lung is allowed to collapse during the operation. These endobronchial tubes are narrower in diameter than are the endotracheal tubes and the design of the cuffs is critical so as to avoid obstruction of the lobar bronchi.

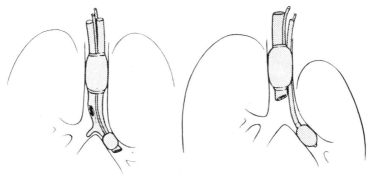

Fig. 8.13 The Carlens double lumen tube. One or other lung can be ventilated independently.

Fig. 8.14 A bronchus blocker in position alongside an endotracheal tube. The left lung is partially collapsed by suction through the blocker.

The administration of an anaesthetic into one lung is of particular value when the other lung is to be removed and there are occasions when the anaesthetist may wish to inflate the lungs independently of one another. For this purpose, double lumen tubes, as for example the Carlens' tube (Fig. 8.13), or Robertshaw's tube may be used.

An alternative technique, used when only part of the lung is to be removed and particularly where there are profuse secretions from the diseased lobe, is to pass a long suction catheter with a cuff at the end into the bronchus supplying the diseased lobe. Such a catheter, known as a bronchus blocker, is shown in Figure 8.14. The blocker is passed through a bronchoscope and positioned accurately; thereafter, the anaesthetic is maintained via an endotracheal tube.

BRONCHOSCOPY

The indications for bronchoscopy in anaesthetic practice are the removal of secretions from the tracheobronchial tree and the removal of foreign bodies from the lungs. One may use a bronchoscope as illustrated in Figure 8.15. The light which illuminates the lumen of the bronchoscope is supplied by a battery stored in the handle in a manner similar to the lighting arrangement for a laryngoscope.

The initial position of the patient's head for bronchoscopy is the same as for laryngoscopy, but thereafter the position must be altered so that the bronchoscope passes readily down the trachea

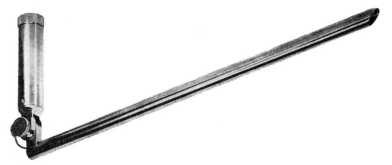

Fig. 8.15 A bronchoscope with battery in the handle suitable for emergency use.

to enter the main bronchi in correct alignment. This involves considerable repositioning of the head and the help of an assistant should be available.

There is a variety of techniques of anaesthesia for bronchoscopy. Local analgesia may be employed without rendering the patient unconscious. A general anaesthetic may be used, anaesthesia being induced with a non-flammable agent such as halothane and the patient is allowed to breathe spontaneously throughout. An alternative is to induce anaesthesia with an intravenous induction agent and thereafter to administer a short-acting myoneural blocking drug such as suxamethonium. Ventilation of the lungs may be continued with a suitable mixture of nitrous oxide and halothane in oxygen admitted through a side arm to the bronchoscope with intermittent occlusion of the proximal end of the instrument to allow inflation of the lungs. Alternatively, a high-pressure injector device may be inserted to the lumen of the bronchoscope to admit oxygen through a venturi device with entrainment of room air in addition. The patient continues to be anaesthetised with intermittent injections of an intravenous anaesthetic and supplementary injections of suxamethonium may be given if required.

9

The prevention and treatment of complications and difficulties during anaesthesia

In addition to watching for signs that the level of anaesthesia is adequate for the surgical operation, the anaesthetist must be prepared to anticipate and prevent, or diagnose and treat, several important complications; some are common, others are rare. Although some complications, such as vomiting and regurgitation, are characteristically associated with the induction of and recovery from anaesthesia, both these and other complications are risks associated with a light level of anaesthesia.

Accidental injection of thiopentone

To an artery. The patient will complain of severe pain or cold at the site of injection perhaps radiating distally. In addition, there may be blanching or a blotchy appearance of the part of the limb normally supplied by the vessel into which the injection has been made. It is essential to leave the needle in position. 20 ml of 0.5 per cent procaine hydrochloride should be injected through it, followed by 40 mg of papaverine in 10 ml of saline; procaine will ease the discomfort and may reduce the degree of vessel spasm while papaverine has a specific vasodilator effect on the smooth muscle of the vessel wall. In the belief that noradrenaline plays a part in this arterial spasm, tolazoline (Priscol) given as a 1 per cent solution (5 ml) has been recommended. However, the relief of arterial spasm and the pain which accompanies it are perhaps of less importance in the long term than the prevention of thrombosis within the vessel. Full anticoagulant therapy with heparin is recommended in the first instance (10 000 units i.m. initially, followed by 5000 units 6-hourly for 48 hours). In addition, oral anticoagulant therapy may be necessary for 2 to 3 weeks after the incident. Obviously, the operation should be postponed whenever possible. If the procedure is of an emergency nature, the consequences of the anticoagulant therapy must be remembered.

A temporary sympathectomy of the limb by blocking either the stellate ganglion or the brachial plexus in its supraclavicular course should be attempted also.

If the veins in the dorsum of the hand and solutions of thiopentone not in excess of 2.5 per cent are used, the risk of this complication will be minimised.

Perivenous. Although solutions of 5 per cent thiopentone caused tissue necrosis in the past, the modern practice of using 2.5 per cent solutions renders this accident less serious. By attention to the technique of intravenous injection (see p. 84), the extravascular injection of more than 1–2 ml of solution will be unlikely. The patient will complain of sharp pain at the site of the injection and an alternative vein should be sought for the purposes of continuing the induction of anaesthesia. As a precaution, 1000 units of hyaluronidase in procaine should be injected into the extravascular deposit of thiopentone. Methohexitone and the non-barbiturate intravenous anaesthetics are not associated with the above risks.

Coughing

This is most likely to cause trouble during an attempted inhalation induction of anaesthesia. It may occur in response to material in the pharynx such as mucus or even gastric contents, in which case, of course, it is a valuable protective reflex. Where it occurs in response to irritant vapours, notably ether, it is still a demonstration of a protective reflex but is now an inconvenience since it delays the smooth uptake of the anaesthetic gas mixture to the lung. The remedy is to reduce the concentration of vapour and to consider the addition of a small quantity of carbon dioxide to the inspired gas. This will stimulate breathing and promote the uptake of the anaesthetic to the lung. Coughing may occur if an oropharyngeal airway is inserted when the level of anaesthesia is too light; the recognition of this cause is usually obvious. On occasions, coughing may complicate the induction of anaesthesia with methohexitone.

Breath-holding

Breath-holding can occur at a light level of anaesthesia and usually signifies that the patient is under the influence of a noxious stimulus to which he may be about to respond. Thus, breath-holding can be caused by irritant inhalation agents and may herald a bout of coughing. Alternatively, a patient who has apparently accepted an inhalation anaesthetic may breath-hold if an oropharyngeal airway is inserted at an unacceptably light level of anaesthesia. Again, coughing may be imminent. At a light level of anaesthesia, a powerful surgical stimulus, such as the incision of the skin or a stretching of the anal canal, may cause breath-holding following a deep inspiration. The addition of carbon dioxide to the inhaled mixture reduces the likelihood of breath-holding, although it is unlikely to be of much value once breath-holding has commenced. Other facets of management include withholding the surgical stimulus and reducing the concentration of the inhalation anaesthetic if this is thought to be irritating. The anaesthetist may be able to limit the period of breath-holding by partially closing the exhaust valve and applying gentle pressure to the anaesthetic reservoir bag, thus gently assisting the anaesthetic mixture towards the lungs. This technique demands experience and skill and we would not wish to give the impression that breath-holding is an indication for vigorous attempts at controlled ventilation. Breath-holding as described here must be distinguished from apnoea as a result of excessively deep anaesthesia or the effects of the myoneural blocking drugs. Making a differential diagnosis includes consideration of the period over which the patient has breathed the anaesthetic gas and the concentrations involved. In light anaesthesia such as would be associated with breath-holding, the respiratory effort up to the moment of cessation will have been vigorous; in these circumstances also, there may be considerable muscle tone, in the airway for example, while the eyelid reflex may be present or the eyes divergent. None of these signs is a feature of deep anaesthesia (see p. 87).

Airway obstruction

During anaesthesia, the airway may be obstructed for many reasons. The commonest is obstruction by the tongue when the

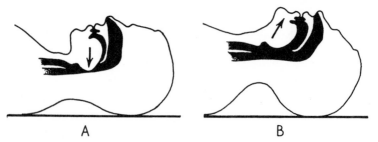

A   B

Fig. 9.1 These figures demonstrate the correct positioning of the head and jaw during anaesthesia and mouth-to-mouth breathing to ensure a clear airway. In A the head is slightly flexed, the jaw is unsupported and the tongue has fallen back obstructing the upper airway. In B the head has been extended, the jaw pulled forward taking the tongue with it and clearing the airway.

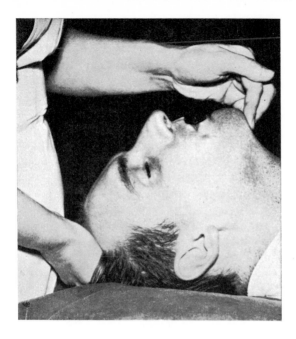

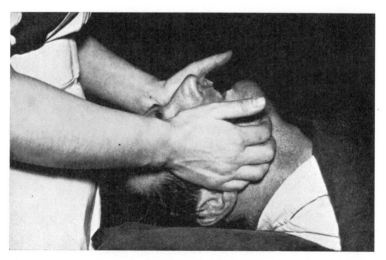

Figs. 9.2 and 9.3 Two alternative methods of supporting the unconscious patient's chin to prevent upper airway obstruction. Whether the tip of the chin or the angles of the jaw are supported the direction of the pull is the same.

muscles which are inserted into its substance lose their tone, thus enabling the tongue to fall towards the posterior wall of the pharynx in a patient who is lying in the supine position. This is accompanied by a noise similar to snoring. The problem is either treated or prevented by supporting the mandible as shown in Figures 9.1, 9.2 and 9.3. Such correct positioning will prevent obstruction by the tongue in the majority of patients who have a well-formed mandible and good natural dentition. In the older patient whose mandible has been eroded by age and in all patients who have no teeth, these manœuvres may not be sufficient on their own. It may be necessary to insert an oropharyngeal airway.

The upper airway may be obstructed by secretions or gastric contents in the pharynx, and in patients with head injuries, blood and cerebrospinal fluid may be present also. Various foreign bodies have been reported as causing obstruction of the upper airway, notably dentures.

The airway may be obstructed also by spasm of the larynx; other causes of laryngeal obstruction are oedema associated with acute infection, particularly in children, tumours of the larynx or epiglottis. The trachea may be narrowed to the point of obstruction as a result of chondromalacia, or following prolonged external compression, for example by a tumour of the thyroid gland.

Laryngeal stridor and spasm
These are common and worrying causes of respiratory obstruction during light anaesthesia. Stridor is caused by an incomplete closure of the vocal cords during inspiration and is characterised by a high-pitched sound during inspiration. In laryngeal spasm, the cords are closed completely; there is no noise because the obstruction is absolute. In both stridor and spasm, there is usually exaggerated activity of the respiratory muscles. These complications may be a result of the irritation of the vocal cords by irritant vapours, unwanted pharyngeal contents, such as vomitus, or solid bodies such as an artificial airway. The ability to produce spasm of the cords is basically a protective reflex. Stridor and spasm may occur also as a result of impulses occurring distant from the larynx, such as incision of the skin or stretching of the anal sphincter.

Sometimes it is claimed that thiopentone, by heightening reflex excitability, may predispose to laryngeal spasm in the presence of irritants. Partial or complete closure of the laryngeal inlet causes hypoxia and retention of carbon dioxide. It is claimed that in healthy patients laryngeal spasm will always 'break' before death ensues because, as the patient becomes grossly hypoxic, the laryngeal muscles weaken and the larynx relaxes. It is unwise to depend on such assumptions, however. In any case, patients who are gravely ill will be placed at serious risk from a prolonged period of laryngeal spasm.

As a first stage in treatment, the source of any irritation should be withdrawn if possible. Thus, if a high concentration of an irritant anaesthetic is being administered, this should be reduced; if an airway has been inserted, this should be withdrawn partially. If it is suspected that fluid has accumulated in the pharynx, the patient's head should be lowered and suction applied to the pharynx. If the stimulus is from the surgical procedure, the surgeon should be asked to wait until the level of anaesthesia has been deepened.

If the closure of the larynx is only partial, that is stridor is present, a high concentration of oxygen should be administered. The particular value of such therapy lies in the fact that reflex spasm is more likely to occur in the presence of hypoxia. If spasm is complete, gentle pressure on the reservoir bag with the exhaust valve almost closed and the circuit filled with oxygen is applied in the hope that the cords will relax momentarily, allowing oxygen to pass to the trachea and lungs. Of course, it is essential during these manœuvres to ensure that the airway above the larynx is clear. If the spasm does not respond to these measures, the anaesthetist will normally administer a short-acting neuromuscular blocking drug such as suxamethonium 50 mg i.v. This will produce complete muscle relaxation and immediate separation of the cords. It is, of course, essential to control ventilation under these circumstances and in most cases it would be appropriate to insert a tracheal tube. Meanwhile, suitable steps should be taken to deepen the level of anaesthesia.

Probably most of the deaths which have occurred as a result of laryngeal spasm could have been prevented if the anaesthetist had followed the simple guidance given in the foregoing. Death from laryngeal spasm is unlikely to occur in experienced hands.

Rarely if a neuromuscular blocking drug is not available and attempts to oxygenate the lungs have failed, a wide-bore needle should be inserted into the trachea through the mid-line at the mid-point of the crico-thyroid membrane. A spontaneously breathing patient will be just able to ventilate the lungs through this narrow channel and oxygen can be added to the air around the hub of the needle. Tracheotomy with a knife is neither necessary nor desirable in the treatment of this complication.

Bronchospasm

Occurring during anaesthesia, this may be mild, associated with a respiratory wheeze, or severe, in which case there may be no appreciable movement of air into and out of the lung and the patient becomes cyanosed very rapidly. There are many causes of bronchospasm, ranging from stimulation of the upper part of the respiratory tract at a light level of anaesthesia, for example in the presence of a tube in the trachea. Bronchospasm may be induced also by the presence of mucus in the respiratory tract. It is claimed that premedication with atropine not only reduces the likelihood of secretions but dilates the bronchial tree also.

Bronchospasm may occur as a result of histamine release following the injection of any one of a number of drugs during anaesthesia. It is probably true to say that none of the drugs given by intravenous injection during anaesthesia is free from the risk of such reactions. Tubocurarine and morphine have a particular reputation in this respect.

A most worrying cause of bronchospasm during anaesthesia is the inhalation of gastric contents (Mendelson's syndrome). This condition is characterised by severe bronchospasm, pulmonary oedema and circulatory failure. The treatment of Mendelson's syndrome is detailed on page 127. Bronchospasm as a result of stimulation of the airway may be helped by the administration of aminophylline 250 mg i.v. and instillation of 3 ml of 4 per cent lignocaine via the endotracheal tube or by direct injection through the crico-thyroid membrane. Chlorpheniramine maleate (Piriton) 10 mg and hydrocortisone 100 mg are recommended in addition in cases of sensitivity to drugs. Because diethylether is a sympathetic stimulant, it has been suggested that controlled ventilation with about 5 per cent of ether in the carrier gas will induce the bronchial musculature to relax. Above all, it is important to ensure that the patient receives a high concentration of oxygen in the inspired gas.

Hiccough

This may be very troublesome, particularly during abdominal surgery. It may also be associated with the injection of methohexitone. The commonest cause, however, is surgical manipulation on the abdominal surface of the diaphragm. A reliable cure for this complication has still to be found, although asking the surgeon to reduce the level of stimulation is often successful. Hiccough may be an indication for deepening the level of anaesthesia, but it should not be regarded as an indication for increasing the dose of a neuromuscular blocking drug. Indeed to do so may result in refractory paralysis at the end of the operation.

Masseter spasm

The masseter muscles are extremely powerful and may develop intense spasm at a light level of anaesthesia, particularly during induction and recovery. This may limit the anaesthetist's access to the mouth and endanger life if there is a need to aspirate material from the pharynx. An additional difficulty arises if an orotracheal tube is in position, because the patient's teeth may obstruct the

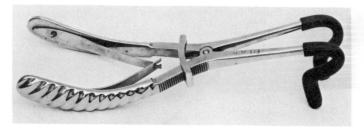

Fig. 9.4 Mouth gag.

tube totally. Although masseter spasm will disappear spontaneously as the level of anaesthesia either lightens or deepens, it may be necessary to give a short-acting myoneural blocking drug to enable the more severe difficulties associated with a masseter spasm to be avoided. On occasion, a gag such as that shown in Figure 9.4 may be employed to force the mouth open; the danger of damage to the teeth from the inexperienced use of this device is considerable.

INADEQUATE VENTILATION

We have considered some of the more dramatic complications which may occur during general anaesthesia. However, equally important is the less dramatic occurrence of inadequate gas exchange which may occur during either spontaneous breathing or controlled ventilation. The problem can be considered under two headings:

1 Inadequacy of alveolar ventilation

In the spontaneously breathing anaesthetised patient, the commonest causes are depression of the respiratory centres which may occur at any stage during the anaesthetic, or partial neuromuscular block as a result of inadequate antagonism of myoneural blockade occurring at the end of anaesthesia or in the early post-operative period. The ventilation may be inadequate in a patient who is undergoing controlled ventilation for which inadequate ventilating volumes have been provided.

For any particular patient, there is a predictable relationship between the amount of the alveolar ventilation, and the alveolar and arterial carbon dioxide tension (Pco_2). This relationship is

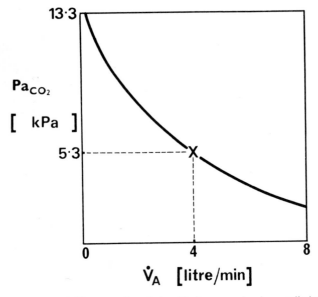

Fig. 9.5 This graph illustrates the relationship between alveolar ventilation ($\dot{V}_A$) and arterial carbon dioxide tension ($Paco_2$).

shown in Figure 9.5; it can be seen that the average aveolar ventilatory requirement to maintain the arterial Pco_2 at the normal value of 5.3 kPa is about 4 l/min. Figure 9.5 shows also that underventilation leads to a rapid increase in the alveolar Pco_2 whereas excessive ventilation (such as may occur as a result of large tidal volumes during controlled ventilation) leads to a reduction in Pco_2.

Normally, when ventilation is reduced carbon dioxide accumulates in the alveolar gas. The combination of a high alveolar CO_2 content and an inadequate supply of oxygen to the alveoli, because of under-ventilation, causes hypoxaemia to co-exist with hypercarbia. However, carbon dioxide may be retained without obvious signs of hypoxaemia if a high concentration of oxygen is given to the patient. This occurs particularly when oxygen is used as the sole carrier gas, for example in the administration of *halothane-in-oxygen anaesthesia*. It is particularly important to appreciate this fact since the agents which are commonly given with oxygen as the sole carrier gas, halothane and cyclopropane, are powerful respiratory depressants.

Inadequate ventilation may be detected by:

Direct measurement of the arterial P_{CO_2}. This is the most reliable index.

Measurement of the respiratory minute volume. This requires an instrument such as the Wright respirometer (Figure 5.3, p. 67). In this case, the patient's basal requirements may be calculated before anaesthesia, from tables such as the Radford nomogram. Alternatively, it may be reasonable to decide that the patient will not be allowed to develop a minute volume less than 5 litre/min. It is important, of course, to remember that it is the *alveolar* minute volume which matters and that the respirometer allows us to measure only the alveolar ventilation and the dead space ventilation combined.

The clinical signs of under-ventilation and of carbon dioxide retention. These signs appear when the arterial P_{CO_2} has reached levels between 10 and 12 kPa and are (a) a hot flushed and moist skin— the so-called boiled lobster syndrome. These signs are caused by dilatation of the arterioles and capillaries by local action of carbon dioxide; (b) the central action of carbon dioxide on the vasomotor centre results in vasoconstriction of the larger vessels, in particular the splanchnic vessels, which results in an increase in arterial pressure; (c) the heart rate increases in the early stages of carbon dioxide retention, although in the later stages the conducting mechanism of the heart is poisoned and the rate slows before the heart fails; (d) the physiological respiratory response to carbon dioxide is an increase in the depth or rate of respiration, or both, but the anaesthetist must not depend too much on these signs since it is often in circumstances in which the patient cannot respond by increasing the rate or depth of respiration that carbon dioxide retention occurs; (e) if the operation has started, there may be an increased oozing from the skin edges; (f) if carbon dioxide retention occurs when the patient is not anaesthetised, for example in the post-operative period, the patient may be seen to be restless and confused.

2. Factors impeding oxygenation of the arterial blood

The most serious problem of oxygenation occurs when the inspired oxygen concentration is less than that in ambient air. The most dramatic example is sudden failure of the oxygen supply to an anaesthetic circuit, with continued supply of nitrous oxide. Such gross asphyxia will lead to circulatory arrest within about 3 minutes.

A more subtle and less dramatic cause of hypoxaemia has been noted in Chapter 2 (p. 23). Under most circumstances of general anaesthesia, there is an increase in the amount of right-to-left shunt across the lung. This is a mixture of both true shunting through discrete non-ventilated channels and of a 'shunt-like' effect (an excess of perfusion in relation to ventilation particularly in the dependent regions of the lung). For practical purposes, the effects of these changes on the arterial Po_2 may be overcome by the administration of not less than 30–40 per cent of oxygen in the inspired gas. However, this statement applies only to patients with normal or near normal cardiorespiratory function. In patients with cyanotic heart disease or with serious lung disease, the maintenance of adequate oxygenation during anaesthesia is one of the major challenges to the anaesthetist. In the most difficult cases, he may have to make intermittent measurements of the arterial Po_2 during and after the operation.

While it is now recognised that during spontaneous breathing with many of the volatile anaesthetics, oxygen tensions below the ideal level and carbon dioxide tensions of almost twice normal have been reached and apparently tolerated by healthy individuals, early recognition of inadequate ventilation is desirable and should be an indication for assisted or controlled ventilation, or an increase in the inspired oxygen concentration as appropriate. Apart from the specific signs associated with hypoxaemia (cyanosis) and carbon dioxide retention (sweating, hypertension, etc.), it is important for all doctors to recognise the abnormal pattern of breathing which is often associated with early respiratory failure. The classic appearance is that of excessive use of the diaphragm in relation to the intercostal muscles. This causes a see-saw type of breathing in which the chest may be drawn in and the abdominal wall protruded during inspiration and vice versa on expiration. Since a jerking movement of the diaphragm occurs also, there may be a tugging action on the mediastinal structures, seen most obviously as a 'tracheal tug'. This effect is most likely to be present in elderly subjects in whom the mediastinum is relatively rigid.

CIRCULATORY COMPLICATIONS

Complications affecting the circulation during anaesthesia may be considered in two main groups. These are (1) changes in arterial pressure and (2) changes in heart rate and rhythm.

1. Changes in arterial pressure

The pressure may decrease, increase or fluctuate widely.

Hypotension

Hypotension may be caused by a variety of factors during anaesthesia. Some of these are associated with central depression of the vasomotor centre, resulting in vasodilatation, some with depression of the myocardium, resulting in a decreased cardiac output, some with diminished venous return to the heart, and others with blood loss.

It is not unusual for a patient, having received premedication, to arrive at the anaesthetic room with an arterial systolic pressure 25 mmHg or more less than the resting level as measured in the ward. This is not an unexpected phenomenon since arterial pressure may decrease by about that amount during normal sleep.

Occasionally, the decrease in pressure is more marked, particularly with some premedicants such as phenothiazine drugs and pethidine. On occasion, marked hypotension may indicate that the patient's functional extracellular fluid volume is abnormally low, such as may occur in hot conditions where there has been profuse sweating or in patients who have suffered peritonitis with considerable loss of fluid into the peritoneal cavity. The administration of thiopentone and many of the techniques which may be used for the maintenance of anaesthesia may cause mild hypotension, particularly before the surgical stimulus has been applied. After surgery has commenced, however, it is common to find the arterial pressure restored to a level not far removed from the resting value.

Prolonged marked hypotension carries the risk of cerebral and myocardial damage from hypoxia or thrombus formation. The oxygenation of these and other tissues does not depend entirely on the level of the arterial pressure. The arterial oxygen content and the blood flow, which varies from organ to organ, and the pooling of blood in dependent parts are all important factors. A further complication, where low blood pressures are maintained for a long period, is that the renal and hepatic circulation may be inadequate with consequent damage to these organs.

The critical mean arterial pressure below which such damage may occur is a matter of some doubt and must be considered in relation to the adequacy of the arterial oxygen availability, although it is widely recognised that renal damage may ensue when the mean pressure falls below 50 mmHg. The critical value may be less than this in some types of deliberately induced arterial hypotension, for example high spinal (subarachnoid) nerve block. However, unless the anaesthetist wishes to reduce the arterial pressure deliberately, it is regarded as good practice to maintain the mean pressure as close as possible to the normal resting value.

Treatment of hypotension
Obviously, this depends on the cause.

1. Where it is thought to be the result of depression by drugs such as halothane, the concentration of the agent should be reduced if possible. As a safeguard, the concentration of oxygen in the inspired gas should be increased. If there is an associated bradycardia (pulse rate less than 55 per min), atropine 0.6 mg i.v. will increase the heart rate and the arterial pressure. The administration of vasopressors is not usually desirable.
2. When ventilation is controlled artificially, the changes in intrathoracic pressure abolish the respiratory pump action which allows the heart and great veins to fill during inspiration. This potentially harmful effect of intermittent positive pressure ventilation is discussed more fully in Chapter 11. In general, however, it is wise to reduce the mean intrathoracic pressure to the lowest possible value consistent with adequate ventilation.
3. Hypotension resulting from loss of blood or extracellular water should be treated by the infusion of blood, plasma, plasma substitutes or the appropriate electrolyte solution (see Ch. 6). Elevation of the legs is an important first aid measure in the treatment of such hypotension.

Hypertension
When this occurs during anaesthesia, it may be a result of underventilation of the lungs with the retention of carbon dioxide and the development of hypoxaemia. The problem has been discussed earlier in this chapter. The treatment may involve the institution of controlled ventilation or an increase in the ventilating volumes, if ventilation is being controlled already.

Hypertension may also occur as a response to the surgical stimulus in a patient who has received inadequate amounts of analgesics. This can be confirmed by looking for other signs of reflex activity and by administering supplementary analgesia, either additional volatile agents to the anaesthetic gas mixture or the intravenous administration of a small dose of a narcotic analgesic.

A rare cause of severe hypertension during anaesthesia is the presence of a phaeochromocytoma.

Hypertension or hypotension are more marked in patients with pre-existing arterial hypertension. Such patients are more susceptible to the cardiovascular effects of drugs, mechanical ventilation and to blood loss. They may also show a marked hypertensive response to inadequate analgesia during surgery.

Changes in heart rate and rhythm

Tachycardia may follow the administration of some drugs used in anaesthesia. It may be a physiological response to hypotension or may be caused by drugs with vagolytic effects, such as atropine, pethidine or gallamine (Flaxedil). Tachycardia may be a sign of excessively light anaesthesia and often accompanies the administration of diethylether as part of the associated sympathomimetic activity.

Whereas tachycardia as a result of the administration of drugs may be accepted, it should be remembered that tachycardia may also be associated with haemorrhage or inadequacy of analgesia or of ventilation. In these circumstances, it is a sign which calls for action to treat the underlying condition.

Bradycardia may occur in association with the administration of cyclopropane or halothane and it is advisable to give atropine as a premedicant before the use of these agents. Even if premedication with atropine has been given, the occurrence of severe bradycardia (55 per minute or less) during anaesthesia with these agents calls for the administration of additional atropine 0.3 to 0.6 mg. Bradycardia may also follow the administration of suxamethonium and may be profound, particularly after a second or subsequent dose. Again, this problem can be minimised by the prophylactic administration of atropine and by restricting the second and further doses of suxamethonium to a maximum of 25 mg.

The administration of hyoscine as a premedicant is sometimes associated with a moderate slowing of the heart rate.

Cardiac arrhythmias of various types occur during anaesthesia and are particularly associated with the administration of halogenated anaesthetics such as chloroform, trichloroethylene and halothane and also with cyclopropane. Many reasons have been advanced for their occurrence but it is now generally agreed that they occur principally when the arterial carbon dioxide tension is high during the administration of these agents. Although it has been shown that arrhythmias are present frequently without any great harm resulting, they should always be considered potentially dangerous and adequate ventilation must be maintained. If this does not cause the arrhythmias to disappear, the concentration of the anaesthetic agent should be reduced or a change be made to another agent.

The arrhythmias may, of themselves, be a sign of severe carbon dioxide retention and oxygen lack.

Where the heart beat is absent and a pulse cannot be felt in a major vessel such as the carotid, a provisional diagnosis of cardiac arrest should be made and confirmatory signs sought (p. 134). It must be stressed that such a diagnosis is made only when pulsation in a major vessel cannot be felt and not when pulsation cannot be obtained in the radial or facial arteries because pulsation in these vessels may be absent during anaesthesia for a variety of reasons, such as pressure of harnesses or vasoconstriction. When the carotid pulse is absent, the apex beat should be checked rapidly by a stethoscope or by palpation. The absence of a heart beat or of pulsation in the major vessel confirms the diagnosis of cardiac arrest.

At this point, a carefully organised plan must be put into effect because, within 3 or 4 minutes of cessation of circulation, irreparable damage to the brain will result. When cardiac massage is instituted, the anaesthetist should ensure that ventilation of the lungs with 100 per cent oxygen is continued throughout the attempts at resuscitation. The problems of cardiac arrest and the methods of dealing with it, both by external cardiac compression and direct cardiac massage, are considered in greater detail in the section dealing with resuscitation (Chapter 12).

So important is it to recognise instantly the occurrence of cardiac arrest that many authorities consider that monitoring of the ECG or the peripheral pulse (by plethysmography), or both, are desirable and on occasion essential. Modern monitoring instruments allow easy display and recording of both features and simple electronic circuits are usually incorporated for the counting of heart rate as a derivative of the ECG or pulse waveform (Fig. 9.6).

Finger plethysmographs have the disadvantage that, during surgery, they tend to pick up extraneous movements of the limb to which they are attached, and during operations when vasoconstriction takes place the record of each beat may be extremely faint. Nevertheless, awareness of vasoconstriction as a result of such findings is useful information in itself.

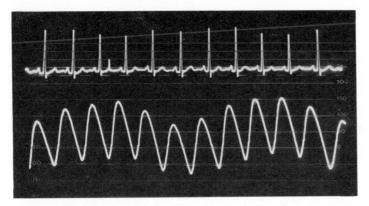

Fig. 9.6 ECG and pulse wave form displayed on an oscilloscope.

Measurement of the central venous pressure via a catheter inserted either into an arm vein or inserted into the external or internal jugular vein, or the subclavian vein, is a popular and useful form of monitoring in the anaesthetised patient undergoing major surgery. Central venous pressure measurements, considered together with other cardiovascular data such as pulse rates and arterial pressure, are a useful indication of the adequacy of blood replacement or the treatment of other fluid losses. In patients with heart failure, however, the interpretation of central venous pressure measurements in relation to fluid loss is difficult. This subject is discussed in greater detail on page 170.

VOMITING AND REGURGITATION

These are particular hazards during induction and recovery, although regurgitation may occur at any time during the maintenance of anaesthesia also.

Vomiting is an active reflex activity involving integrated action of the respiratory muscles, the larynx and the vomiting and respiratory centres in the medulla. It is worth emphasising that the process cannot occur unless there is such a degree of reflex integrity that the patient will be conscious and the cough reflex will be present. Thus, the risk to the respiratory tract is much less than in the case of regurgitation.

Regurgitation is the result of the intragastric pressure being sufficiently great to overcome the competence of the sphincter-like protective mechanisms at the lower end of the oesophagus. Thus, regurgitation can occur both in the enfeebled conscious patient and also in the unconscious and it constitutes a serious risk that the regurgitated material will spill over into the respiratory tract.

The risk of vomiting and regurgitation is so great that anaesthesia should not be undertaken in a patient who is known to have food in his stomach unless the indications for operation are extremely urgent. The normal emptying time of the stomach is somewhere between 4 and 5 hours. This may be hastened by the use of a drug such as metoclopramide (Maxolon) 20 mg i.v., and may be delayed following the ingestion of a fatty meal or as a consequence of injury.

Various manoeuvres have been introduced to promote the emptying of the stomach before anaesthesia is undertaken in an emergency. These include the insertion of tubes for the aspiration of stomach contents or the administration of apomorphine to induce vomiting. Quite apart from the barbaric nature of these measures, they are unacceptable because they cannot be guaranteed to be effective.

The treatment of vomiting and regurgitation is to lower the patient's head and turn it to one side; the vomitus should be aspirated from the pharynx. During light anaesthesia, this may be all that is required and if the anaesthetic is continued with the head down and to the side, regurgitated material is unlikely to pass into the trachea. If inhalation of vomitus has taken place, steps should be taken to aspirate the trachea immediately, either through an endotracheal tube or by bronchoscopy. The use of a head-down posture may assist these measures.

Sellick's manoeuvre. If an assistant applies firm pressure on the cricoid cartilage with his thumb and index finger (Fig. 9.7), this will occlude the oesophagus and is probably the most effective precaution which can be taken to prevent regurgitated stomach contents from reaching the laryngeal inlet.

The insertion of a cuffed tracheal tube as early as possible in the conduct of an anaesthetic will not prevent vomiting or regurgitation, but will play a major part in ensuring that the gastric contents do not reach the bronchial tree. It is foolish to assume, however, that cuffed tubes offer total protection; the cuff may rupture or its seal with the trachea may be inadequate.

If gastric contents enter the respiratory tract, attempts should be made to remove the material as rapidly as possible by suction with a fine catheter through a tracheal tube. If the quantity is considerable, or the pH of the contents irrespective of quantity is very low, there is a risk of the development of aspiration pneumonitis

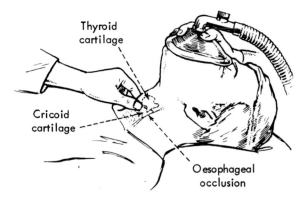

Fig. 9.7 Firm pressure on the cricoid by an assistant during induction of anaesthesia may prevent regurgitation of stomach contents by occluding the oesophagus.

(Mendelson's syndrome), characterised by acute bronchospasm and by circulatory collapse. The mortality from Mendelson's syndrome is difficult to measure but may amount to about 25 per cent of all patients who develop the condition. The lungs should be artificially ventilated with oxygen-enriched air, and antispasmodic agents such as aminophylline and hydrocortisone should be given intravenously. In addition, support of the circulation by the administration of plasma is important.

MALIGNANT HYPERPYREXIA

This is the name given to a syndrome whose main features are increased muscle tone and high fever. While it may occur in association with any inhalation anaesthetic, it is seen most often when suxamethonium or halothane have been used. The incidence varies in different populations but is quoted as 1 in 100 000 anaesthetics. It is associated with an inherited abnormality which may be revealed by abnormal levels of the serum concentration of creatine phosphokinase (CPK) or by muscle biopsy. It is suggested that the condition may be associated with various myopathies occasionally manifest as an inguinal hernia or strabismus in a child.

Treatment is directed towards lowering the body temperature, and correcting the metabolic acidosis and hyperkalaemia which develop. Dexamethasone 100 mg i.v. has been recommended. The lungs should be ventilated with a high concentration of oxygen.

The necessary ventilation pressures may be extremely high in view of increased tone in the respiratory muscles.

Mortality from the condition is high and all relatives of a susceptible patient should be screened with a view to preventing a similar occurrence at a later date. Careful interpretation of CPK values with biochemical advice, perhaps muscle biopsy for *in vitro* examination of the effects of various anaesthetics on the muscle specimen, and correlation with previous anaesthetic experiences have been advised.

Any subsequent operations upon survivors or their families should be conducted under general anaesthesia in which thiopentone, the non-depolarising myoneural blocking drugs, oxygen, nitrous oxide, and narcotic analgesics such as morphine or phenoperidine are the only agents employed. In spite of this, there is one report of malignant hyperpyrexia having been triggered by exposure to nitrous oxide. It should be emphasised that susceptibility to malignant hyperpyrexia is a contra-condition to the use of local anaesthetic drugs, especially lignocaine which are thought to be able to trigger the condition also.

10

Recovery room—after care of patients

All patients should be observed during the post-operative period, ideally in a centralised recovery room beside the operating theatre. The length of stay in this room will depend on the condition of the patient and the nature of the surgical procedure and anaesthesia. Close observation and care of patients during the crucial post-operative period when consciousness and reflexes may still be impaired results in economy of nursing and medical personnel and apparatus. Where such facilities are not available some compromise is necessary but it should be possible to nurse major surgical, seriously ill and emergency cases through the recovery period in a side ward near the theatre or in a screened-off section of the general ward. Whatever the local arrangement, it is essential that all nurses and medical staff engaged in post-operative care should be trained specially for this work and be capable of carrying out certain emergency resuscitative measures.

COMPLICATIONS OF ANAESTHESIA

The complications requiring the special attention of the recovery room staff readily fall into five groups:

Respiratory: Obstruction of the airway; respiratory inadequacy and respiratory arrest.

Circulatory: Hypotension; cardiac irregularities and cardiac arrest.

Gastro-intestinal: Vomiting and regurgitation of stomach contents.

Renal: The development of acute reversible intrinsic renal failure (acute tubular necrosis).

Neurological sequelae.

These main groups may frequently overlap; for example a patient while still recovering from anaesthesia may regurgitate, inhale gastric contents and suffer respiratory obstruction. Untreated, this could lead to cardiac arrest and death.

We will now consider these complications in more detail, describing their mechanism, their recognition and appropriate treatment.

Respiratory complications

Obstruction of the airway

The commonest respiratory complication, in the immediate postoperative period, is obstruction of the patient's upper airway. The three commonest causes are: the tongue falling back against the posterior wall of the pharynx when the patient is supine; the presence of foreign material in the pharynx; and laryngeal spasm. Respiratory obstruction can again be diagnosed when movements of the chest and abdomen are exaggerated but very little air passes through the nose or mouth with the patient becoming increasingly cyanosed. Laryngeal spasm often produces a 'crowing' noise as air passes through the constricted larynx. It is worth remembering that *noisy breathing is always obstructed breathing, but not all obstructed breathing is noisy.*

Treatment. Secure a clear airway immediately. This is usually accomplished by pulling the lower jaw upwards and forwards, thus pulling the tongue away from the posterior pharyngeal wall. Only rarely should it be necessary to grip the tongue and pull it forward with forceps. Suction may be required to remove any obstruction, for example mucus. Oxygen may have to be administered but is quite useless unless the airway is already clear.

If no improvement follows these manœuvres GET HELP quickly.

Respiratory insufficiency

Despite an unobstructed upper airway, some patients may not breathe deeply enough to ensure adequate respiratory exchange in the alveoli. Any interference with this mechanism results in hypoxia and carbon dioxide accumulation (Figs 9.5 and 10.1). This may occur for many reasons:

Obstruction of the smaller airways or bronchi.
Depression of the respiratory centre following head injuries or cerebrovascular accidents, or the prolonged effects of anaesthetic agents.

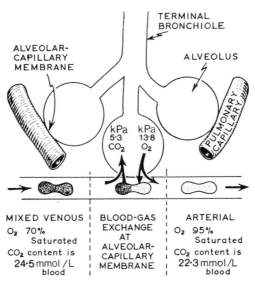

Fig. 10.1 The alveolar-capillary diagram: this diagram demonstrates the blood-gas changes which take place during normal respiration as the blood passes through the lungs.

Disease of or damage to the nervous pathways to the muscles of respiration, for example poliomyelitis.

Weakness of the muscles of respiration as in myasthenia gravis, or when the action of relaxant drugs has not been fully reversed at the end of the operation.

Removal of lung tissue, as in lobectomy or pneumonectomy.

Pre-existing lung disease, for example bronchitis or emphysema.

Constriction of the chest wall or abdomen interfering with normal expansion during breathing. This may be the result of pre-existing disease of the thoracic cage, for example ankylosing spondylitis, or a simpler cause sometimes found is the application of too tight a dressing following operation. The recognition of inadequate respiration has already been discussed (p. 117).

If the patient has previously been conscious, respiratory inadequacy may be evidenced by increasing restlessness, confusion, drowsiness and eventual coma.

Treatment. Having secured a clear airway, the next step, no matter what the underlying cause of the respiratory inadequacy, must always be to assist the patient's own inadequate efforts. Increasing the amount of oxygen in the inspired air alone rarely results in improvement. Many simple devices are now available to augment the patient's ventilation. These enable the doctor or nurse to administer atmospheric air or oxygen by intermittent compression of a bag or bellows, for example Ambu resuscitator (Fig. 10.2).

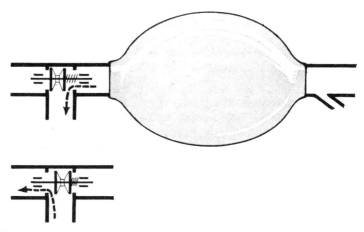

Fig. 10.2 The Ambu resuscitator: additional oxygen may be fed into the bag through the small side tube at the right of the picture, thus enriching the air which is driven into the patient's lungs when the bag is compressed. On the left of the illustration is the non-return valve connected to a mask or endotracheal tube by the vertical limb. The patient's expirations are delivered to the atmosphere through the horizontal limb of the valve.

No recovery room should be without one or other of these simple devices and all staff should be skilled in their use. When apparatus is not immediately available the physician must resort to other measures to support the patient's failing or absent ventilation. The simplest and most effective of these is the technique of expired air resuscitation or mouth-to-mouth breathing. A detailed description of this method is given in Chapter 12.

Circulatory complications

When considering *circulatory changes* following anaesthesia, it is important to remember the significance of alterations in the patient's colour. Pallor or flushing in the absence of other signs of shock or of inadequate respiration, may be quite normal. Cyanosis *always* calls for urgent treatment.

The temperature of patients returning to a recovery room postoperatively may often be found to be slightly sub-normal. While it is important to prevent such patients shivering, only exceptionally should heat be applied, as this results in diversion of the blood from the vital organs to the skin.

Pulse

The pulse rate should be carefully observed during the immediate post-operative period.

A moderate tachycardia (80–100/min) commonly follows major surgery but a persistent tachycardia, particularly if it is increasing, should always be regarded as a danger sign, indicating perhaps haemorrhage or inadequate respiration.

Arterial pressure

Following a major operation the arterial pressure may be below the pre-operative value, as a result of the surgery itself and of the continuing action of drugs administered by the anaesthetist. A systolic pressure of about 20 mmHg below the pre-operative value can often be accepted, but where it continues to fall or to rise unduly an explanation should be sought. All patients who have had a general anaesthetic, and some to whom a regional analgesic has been given, are liable to hypotension and even sudden cardiac arrest if they are roughly handled or put in the sitting-up position (postural hypotension); they should be moved gently from trolley to bed and kept flat (or in the tonsillar position) until recovery is complete. In special cases, the bed may be tilted to a moderate head-down position for the first hour or two.

Frequent arterial pressure readings are time consuming and not usually necessary (for example not more often than every 20–30 minutes). Close observation of colour change in the skin, level of consciousness and pulse rate provide the necessary information in most patients.

There are some patients for whom continuous arterial pressure recording during anaesthesia and throughout the recovery period is necessary. This is common after major cardiothoracic procedures or following surgery and anaesthesia in patients with severe multiple injuries. Accurate and continuous measurement of arterial pressure is achieved in this situation by means of an indwelling arterial cannula coupled to a pressure transducer system with the resulting signal displayed on an oscilloscope or pen-recorder.

Venous pressure

The measurement of central venous pressure is frequently made by the anaesthetist in theatre, particularly in cases of severe injuries or during surgery involving a large loss of blood. The central venous pressure is a sensitive index of changes in circulating blood volume and begins to fall before changes in pulse rate or systemic arterial pressure can be detected. Measurements may continue to be made during the recovery period as a guide to further blood or plasma requirements. In certain circumstances measurement of central venous pressure can be misleading because of previous cardiac or pulmonary disease, and pressure recordings from the left side of the heart more truly reflect the performance of the heart as a pump. A flow-directed catheter (Swan–Ganz catheter) can be passed via the superior vena cava through the right atrium and ventricle and allowed to wedge in a branch of the pulmonary artery. The pulmonary 'wedge' pressure measured in this way is nearly identical to the left atrial pressure and changes in its value can provide a more precise guide for the clinician as to the need for further intravenous infusions or the administration of cardiac drugs such as digitalis when there is evidence of a failing heart action.

Cardiac arrest

Cardiac irregularities in the post-operative period should always be reported to the anaesthetist. Atrial fibrillation in elderly patients may occur following major surgery and its onset is often accompanied by a fall in blood pressure. Bursts of extrasystoles (dropped-beats) may herald the onset of ventricular fibrillation and cardiac arrest. The precise diagnosis of cardiac irregularities usually depends on the ECG and therefore the earlier their occurrence is reported the better.

The most sudden and dramatic of all emergencies with which the recovery room personnel may have to deal is that of cardiac arrest. This may follow untreated respiratory inadequacy or a period of persistent hypotension due to any cause, but it can frequently occur without warning. Any patients who are especially at risk, for example those with some degree of heart-block pre-operatively, should be indicated to the staff by the anaesthetist. In healthy adults, the sensitive tissue of the brain will only survive the results of circulatory standstill and acute hypoxia for a period of about 3 minutes. The immediate recognition of this condition is therefore of the utmost importance if resuscitation is to be successful.

Signs of 'apparent cardiac arrest'. The term 'apparent cardiac arrest' is used deliberately since, if the cardiac action and circulation are so poor that the following signs are present, then immediate treatment is required even if the heart has not quite stopped.

There are three signs:
— *Pallor or cyanosis of the skin,* that is a sudden deterioration of the skin colour.

— *Absence of palpable carotid pulses in the neck*. N.B. not the radial pulses as these are often difficult to feel.
— *Rapidly dilating pupils*. This is a most reliable sign of cerebral hypoxia.

Two secondary signs should be noted.

— *Loss of consciousness*. This, of course, applies only if the patient was not already unconscious.
— *Cessation of respiration*. If action is not taken quickly enough following cardiac arrest then respiratory arrest will follow.

Treatment of cardiac arrest. If these signs are present, *immediate action* is required. Until recently this would have taken the form of direct cardiac massage but, since 1960, a new method of indirect or external cardiac compression is to be preferred, in the first instance. This method may only fill the gap in time until direct massage can be instituted or may actually itself be sufficient to restore cardiac action and circulation completely. The technique of external cardiac compression is described in Chapter 12.

Gastro-intestinal complications

It is necessary to distinguish between vomiting which is an active process and regurgitation which is a passive and more insidious complication. Regurgitation is seldom accompanied by any outward signs or sounds and occurs when the patient is at a deeper level of unconsciousness and his cough reflex is absent or less active than normal. Unless adequate precautions have been taken inhalation of the gastric contents will certainly occur. The vomiting patient on the other hand can usually cough vigorously and the vomitus unless excessive in quantity can be expelled without danger of inhalation.

This complication is most likely to occur if the stomach has not been emptied adequately before operation, if there was vomiting pre-operatively, or if the nature of the illness results in delayed gastric emptying.

Certain anaesthetic agents predispose to nausea and vomiting in the post-operative period, for example cyclopropane and diethylether, but with modern anaesthetic techniques vomiting from this latter cause is uncommon.

Inhalation of gastric contents can result in sudden death from drowning or in acute hypoxia from laryngeal or bronchial spasm. A late result may be the development of pulmonary collapse, pneumonia or lung abscess. One group of patients, in whom inhalation of foreign material is particularly likely, deserves special mention. When the pharynx and vocal cords have been anaesthetised by topical application of an analgesic agent, for example lignocaine 4 per cent, to facilitate endoscopy, the loss of sensation often exceeds the actual operating time by up to two hours. Thus fluids or solids must not be given until the analgesic has ceased to act, lest they are inhaled when the patient attempts to swallow. A simple label on the patient's forehead, indicating that a topical analgesic has been used, is a useful precaution.

Treatment. The best treatment of the condition is prevention. Wherever possible, the stomach should be empty pre-operatively. Even when a gastric tube is left in place after operation, regurgitation may still take place alongside the tube, particularly if drainage is not free, for example if a clamp or spigot is left on the upper end of the tube.

The dangers of regurgitation may be prevented to a large extent by correct posturing of the patient in bed, that is the tonsillar position (Fig. 7.4).

If regurgitation does occur:

1. *Keep the head low.* This ensures that all the material will flow out of the mouth and not enter the respiratory tract.

2. *Clear the mouth and pharynx* with swabs or suction.

3. Having cleared the airway, *ensure that respiration is adequate.* If cyanosis persists, administer oxygen.

4. If there is evidence that stomach contents have been inhaled more active measures are indicated. Acute pulmonary oedema may follow inhalation of even a small quantity of acid material and should be treated with oxygen, assistance to ventilation, steroid therapy and antibiotics.

Renal complications

It has been said that one unnecessary risk to the critically ill patient could be avoided if as much attention was paid to measurement of urine flow as to changes in pulse rate. Normally functioning kidneys are essential not only to body water and electrolyte balance but also to acid–base homeostasis. Incipient renal failure may pass unnoticed in the immediate post-operative period unless there is a proper understanding of its mechanisms and a recognition of the 'high risk' situations in which it is likely to occur.

A simple classification of renal failure is:

Pre-renal—where there is severe dehydration or loss of circulatory blood volume.

Intrinsic—where the renal tissue itself suffers damage which may or may not be reversible.

Post-renal—for example where bilateral calculi obstruct the ureters.

We are concerned here only with the pre-renal and intrinsic types. In the pre-renal type of failure which is commonly met with in the surgical patient, treatment consists of adequate restoration of the circulating blood volume, replacement of fluids and correction of electrolyte deficiencies. This will usually result in a return of normal urine flow from the previous oliguric state. Uncorrected or undetected, the pre-renal type of failure can progress to the intrinsic variety which has in times past been referred to as acute tubular necrosis. Failure to secure a normal urine flow (*at least 30 ml per hour in the adult*) following restoration of the circulating blood volume may indicate that intrinsic failure is already established. Even at this stage the situation may be reversible if a diuretic such as 20 per cent mannitol is given intravenously. Failure to respond to this therapy is an indication for further treatment by the renal physicians which may be conservative or may consist of repeated peritoneal dialysis or haemodialysis until normal renal function returns.

To summarise, the predisposing factors are:

— Reduced renal blood flow due to a reduction in circulating blood, plasma or water and electrolytes.
— Metabolic acidosis which, for example, is almost invariably present in the shocked patient.
— Excessive circulating haemoglobin or myoglobin as commonly found in grave multiple injuries.
— Sepsis.
— Surgery on the aorta at or above the level of the renal vessels.

Close observation of these patients in the immediate post-operative phase is essential and should consist of hourly urine volume measurement along with blood pressure and central venous pressure measurements. Frequent blood-gas analysis to detect any metabolic acidosis is important, as are the measurement of urine and plasma osmolalities. The ratio of urine to plasma osmolality (milliosmoles per kg) taken in conjunction with hourly urine flow is a valuable diagnostic measure in the detection of early acute reversible intrinsic renal failure (acute tubular necrosis) and its differentiation from pre-renal failure. A ratio of more than 2:1

denotes the pre-renal variety while a ratio progressively less than 1.7 : 1 indicates early to established intrinsic renal failure.

The initial treatment is outlined below but the early recognition of the condition and collaboration with the renal physicians is of the first importance.

Treatment. Maintenance of normal blood volume.
Correction of fluid and electrolyte deficiencies.
100 ml of 20 per cent mannitol intravenously (two or three doses maximum).

Neurological sequelae
Although neurological complications of anaesthesia are relatively rare it is important to recognise their occurrence. Many are preventable if due care and attention are paid to the preparation of the patient for anaesthesia and intra-operative management. The following are some examples of this type of complication.

1. Cerebral damage: due to prolonged hypotension or other causes of cerebral hypoxia.
2. Drug-induced damage: Trigeminal paralysis following inhalation of toxic degradation products of trichloroethylene if the latter has been used in conjunction with sodalime in a closed anaesthetic circuit. Lower motor neurone lesions in patients with unrecognised porphyria who have been given certain drugs such as barbiturates.
3. Direct damage to nerve tissue: this can follow a subarachnoid injection where the spinal cord is injured by the needle.

Damage to the median nerve at the antecubital fossa can occur if an intravenous injection of an irritant drug, for example sod. thiopentone, is misplaced.

Direct pressure damage to cranial and peripheral nerves can occur if care is not taken with the positioning of a patient on the operating table, or anaesthetic tubing etc. is not adequately padded, for example supraorbital nerve and lateral popliteal nerve.

CARE OF SPECIAL CASES IN THE RECOVERY ROOM

There are additional points to observe in the management of patients who have undergone certain special types of surgery or anaesthesia.

Epidural and subarachnoid analgesia
These analgesic techniques interfere with three important func-

tions of the patient's normal defence mechanism and this state of affairs often persists well into the recovery period.

Analgesia

The regions of the body, and particularly the skin, served by the nerves which have been blocked as they leave the subarachnoid (spinal) or epidural spaces, may still be partially or completely affected post-operatively. So far as the skin is concerned the patient will not respond normally to pain, heat or cold. Contact with a rough projection on the bed or a hot-water bottle will therefore result in injury (traumatic ulceration or burns).

Reflexes

The normal postural reflexes will be depressed. These reflexes normally prevent over-stretching of muscles or over-extension of joints. Damage can result if the limbs are allowed to remain in abnormal positions for long periods.

The use of ripple mattresses is of great assistance in the prevention of bed sores in any patient where the one posture is, of necessity, maintained for a long time. An alternative to the ripple mattress is the medical sheepskin which supports the patient on a cushion of air trapped among the fibres of the material.

Sympathetic blockade

Under sympathetic blockade the normal control of the peripheral blood vessels which helps to maintain the blood pressure at the normal levels is temporarily lost. Thus, blood pools in the dependent parts of the body and a severe fall in blood pressure occurs. Therefore, patients under the influence of a spinal or epidural analgesic must be nursed in the recumbent position and occasionally in the head-down position until the normal tone returns to the cardiovascular system.

There are other points to observe in the management of such cases:

Headache. Not infrequently this follows subarachnoid analgesia and its causation is obscure. However, it is well known that headache is much commoner in patients who have not been nursed in the supine position for at least 12 hours after the operation.

Acute retention of urine. This can occur particularly in older men with prostatic enlargement. However, while the analgesic effect persists, the distended bladder does not cause undue discomfort. The abdomen therefore should be examined regularly for any sign of bladder distension, and catheterisation may be required.

Sterility. Particular care must be taken of patients in whom a continuous epidural analgesia is being maintained post-operatively. The staff may be instructed to make the intermittent injections at certain intervals and *absolute* sterility is essential.

Induced hypotensive anaesthesia

Some surgical procedures are facilitated if bleeding in the field of operation is reduced to a minimum by lowering the blood pressure deliberately during anaesthesia, for example brain surgery, micro-surgery of the middle ear and plastic surgery. Hypotension may be induced in one of two ways:

1. By epidural or subarachnoid analgesia.
2. By the intravenous injection of ganglion blocking drugs such as trimetaphan (Arfonad).

The loss of vasomotor tone (that is dilatation of the blood vessels) produced by these methods may last well into the recovery phase and although the patient may have become fully conscious, he is still very likely to suffer a severe fall in blood pressure if allowed to sit up. Frequent pulse and blood pressure recording is therefore of the greatest importance in these patients, until the hypotensive effect wears off.

Induced hypothermia

This technique is usually confined to cardiovascular and neurosurgical procedures, or following severe head injuries. The patient's body temperature is lowered to between 29°C and 32°C (normal body temperature 37°C) and active rewarming of such cases is carried out in the recovery room until the body temperature is about 36°C. Rewarming is carried out with electric blankets, special mattresses which contain circulating warm water, or by a fan blowing warm air over the body surface. Although the process is always closely supervised by the anaesthetist, the recovery room staff has an important part to play. The recording of temperature at frequent intervals, in addition to heart rate, arterial pressure and respiratory rate, is usually the responsibility of the nurse. A few words of explanation about temperature recording in these cases may be useful at this point.

'Body' temperature is a meaningless phrase unless the site at which the recording is made is indicated, for example rectum, oesophagus, nasopharynx or axilla. Commonly during rewarming

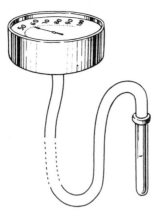

Fig. 10.3 A rectal thermometer. The sensing device is a reservoir bulb filled with mercury. This is connected to the gauge by a flexible capillary tube. The probe is left *in situ* and frequent readings can be made.

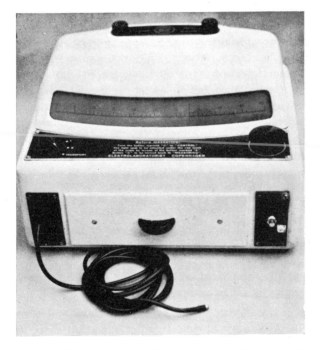

Fig. 10.4 A recording thermometer with an oesophageal lead attached.

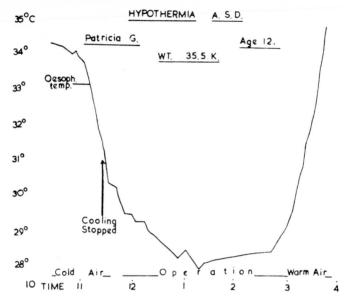

Fig. 10.5 This temperature chart shows the oesophageal temperature changes during the repair of an atrial septal defect (ASD) in a child weighing 35.5 kg.

the rectal or oesophageal temperature is monitored by specially designed continuously recording thermometers (Figs 10.3 and 10.4). The mercury clinical thermometer is not suitable. The temperature is read at frequent intervals, for example five minutes until a return to normal is achieved. Figure 10.5 shows the changes in oesophageal temperature in a patient, during the whole preoperative cooling procedure and the post-operative warming phase.

Special attention must be paid to the skin during rewarming to avoid contact burns and pressure sores.

Endoscopy
The diagnostic procedures of laryngoscopy, bronchoscopy and oesophagoscopy are frequently carried out under topical analgesia, with or without a general anaesthetic as well. Lignocaine in a 4 per cent solution is commonly employed and its analgesic action may last up to two hours. During this period there is a loss of sensation in the mouth, oropharynx and larynx and the cough reflex is depressed. It is obvious that two dangers must be avoided in the recovery room:

— Any solids or liquids given orally may enter the lungs.
— Hot liquids may cause burns to the anaesthetised area.

For a period of at least three hours from the start of anaesthesia, no fluids or solids are given to these patients despite the fact that they may be fully conscious and co-operative.

Due to the absence of the cough reflex, secretions tend to accumulate in the mouth and airway and patients must be encouraged to cough them up or, if necessary, they must be removed by gentle suction. The use of the tonsillar position in bed, even when the patient is fully conscious, has much to recommend it.

Restless patients

Restlessness, during recovery from anaesthesia, is common and the diagnosis and treatment of the underlying cause is worthy of mention. Too often such restlessness is interpreted only as a need for a sedative or analgesic. It is essential that the cause be accurately identified and sedation must be withheld until this has been done. The following are some of the possible causes of post-operative restlessness:

Inadequate ventilation. This can be diagnosed with certainty if signs of hypoxia or carbon dioxide retention are present (pp. 119 and 120).

Haemorrhage. A fall in arterial pressure with tachycardia is strongly suggestive of hidden bleeding.

Pain other than wound pain. This may result from a full bladder, pins in the dressings puncturing the skin, contact with hot-water bottles, etc.

When other causes have been excluded, and only then, is it safe to assume that pain at the site of the operation is responsible and an analgesic is indicated, for example morphine 10–15 mg. Occasionally, in the absence of pain, a sedative to allay nervousness is sufficient, for example lorazepam 2–4 mg or diazepam 10 mg.

Post-thoracotomy

Certain post-operative complications may occur in patients who have undergone thoracotomy. The two most dangerous are unrecognised bleeding inside the chest resulting in a *haemothorax*, and air inside the chest escaping from a damaged area of lung resulting in *pneumothorax*. The presence of blood or air in quantity within the pleural cavity causes collapse of the underlying lung resulting in inadequate ventilation. Because of these dangers a drain is usually inserted by the surgeon into the pleural cavity at the end of the operation. If this were an ordinary tube drain such as is commonly used following abdominal surgery, air would be sucked into the chest during inspiration and the lung would collapse.

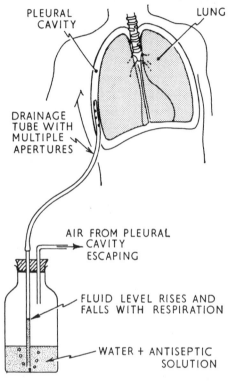

Fig. 10.6 Water-seal drain: It is important that the chest drain be attached to the glass tube which opens under the surface of the liquid in the bottle.

There are three variations of the water-sealed drain in common use. The first of these is illustrated in Figure 10.6 and is the method most commonly employed. Where large quantities of blood or fluid are expected, a second collecting bottle can be interposed between the water-seal bottle and the patient. This enables a more precise measurement of the blood loss to be made when the collecting bottle is suitably calibrated.

The third method of drainage is used in situations where it is desirable to be able to control the negative pressure within the water-sealed system to keep the lung fully expanded (Fig. 10.7).

This time the second bottle is on the opposite side of the water-sealed bottle from the patient and has an additional tube open to atmosphere at one end and submerged 5 to 10 cm below the surface of the sterile liquid at the other. Adjustment of this tube at different depths below the surface maintains the negative pressure within the whole system at -5 to -10 cm H_2O when the bottle outlet is attached to suction apparatus and this is usually done where there is a large air-leak from the lung such as is encountered in bronchopleural fistula. The application of a dangerously large negative pressure to the pleural cavity is avoided since if the -5 to -10 cm selected pressure is exceeded, air will be drawn into the system from the atmosphere via the open end of the third tube.

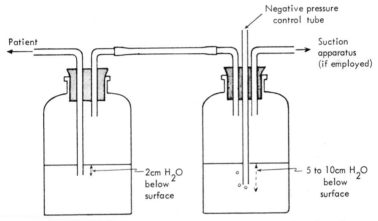

Fig. 10.7 A water-seal system enabling the negative pressure to be adjusted as required.

When suction is used in this way, air should always be seen to be bubbling gently from the submerged end of the tube.

Although the intrathoracic catheter is generally inserted so that it lies in the lower part of the pleural cavity when blood and fluid is being drained, an apical drain is best where air is leaking from the lung. The reason for employing the higher position is that air collects in the upper pleural cavity if the patient is semi-recumbent or erect.

A word of warning is necessary. During transportation of the patient or moving him about in bed the bottle must always be kept at a lower level than the chest, unless the tubing is clamped, otherwise the fluid in the bottle will flow back up the tube into the chest. If the chest drain is patent the level of the fluid in the descending glass tube will fluctuate smoothly with respiration. If it does not,

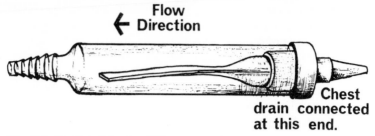

Fig. 10.8 The Heimlich valve: This one-way valve is interposed between the chest drain and the drainage bottle. Air and blood may flow in the direction indicated but the rubber valve prevents air entering the pleural cavity.

then the tube is probably blocked with debris or clotted blood and must be gently 'milked' until patent again. Alternatively, a one-way valve may be attached to the chest drain (Fig. 10.8).

Although a chest drain is usually introduced to the pleural cavity formally during open thoracotomy there are occasions in emergency situations where a catheter has to be introduced quickly by a 'blind' technique. This is done where there has been a rapid and dangerous accumulation of air or blood in the pleural cavity often after an injury to the chest. The catheter may be placed at the base or the apex of the cavity and this is done usually under local analgesia, by means of a trocar which is inserted within the catheter. Through a small skin incision the trocar and catheter

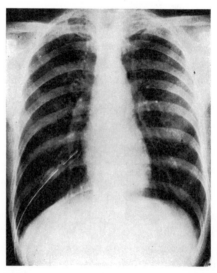

Fig. 10.9 An Argyle thoracic catheter in position showing the radio-opaque marker.

are advanced between the ribs until the pleural cavity is pene-
trated. The trocar is then removed and the catheter connected to
the water-seal drainage bottle in the usual way. In order to facilitate positioning of the catheter it has a radio-opaque strip along
its length which enables it to be seen clearly on X-ray (Fig. 10.9).

Patients who have had a thoracic operation may have considerable wound pain and pleural irritation from the chest drain. This
discourages them from moving, breathing deeply or coughing. Of
course, this results in retention of secretions in the bronchi and
leads to hypoxia and carbon dioxide retention. Adequate doses of
analgesics must be given to permit a good respiratory effort to be
maintained and coughing must be encouraged to clear the airway
of secretions. Nowhere is the value of the post-operative recovery
room more apparent than in the supervision of these patients.

After craniotomy
The intensive care of patients who have undergone neurosurgical
procedures is worthy of special mention. These patients may be
conscious or unconscious. In the case of the conscious patient the
problem usually resolves itself into the careful observation of the
conscious level, the cardiopulmonary state and the ensuring of
adequate nutrition. Where the patient is unconscious, meticulous
attention must be paid to alterations in the level of consciousness
and for this purpose a special chart is of assistance. Signs of increased intracranial pressure are an indication for urgent intervention to avoid irreparable cerebral damage from 'coning'. The
measurement of central venous pressure is invaluable as an uncontrolled increase can result in increased intracranial pressure.

The management of the airway in those patients is of paramount
importance since hypoxia or retention of carbon dioxide can increase cerebral oedema and prejudice recovery. The use of nasotracheal tubes is of great assistance here and reduces the need for
tracheostomy. Active cooling measures may be required where
hyperthermia is a complication.

INHALATION THERAPY

The gas most commonly utilised in inhalation therapy is oxygen,
although mixtures of oxygen with carbon dioxide (in carbon monoxide poisoning) or helium (in respiratory obstruction) are used
occasionally. Increasing the concentration of oxygen, even to 100
per cent, in the inspired gas or air is of limited value if respiratory
obstruction or inadequate respiration is present. Where hypoxia

is present and oxygen therapy instituted the person who orders this treatment must ensure that the airway is clear and ventilation adequate—or he should seek help. Delivering 100 per cent oxygen to the face of an apnoeic patient without ensuring a clear airway, and assisting ventilation manually or mechanically is futile.

Rationale of oxygen therapy

Ambient air contains approximately 21 per cent of oxygen at a partial pressure of about 20 kPa. When a patient breathes 100 per cent oxygen the nitrogen in the lungs is 'washed' out and the partial pressure of oxygen in the lungs is increased to nearly 80–85 kPa. Thus the pressure gradient for diffusion of oxygen across the alveolar–capillary membrane is increased greatly, more oxygen is dissolved in the plasma and the plasma content is increased approximately sevenfold. It is apparent that any further increase in the plasma content of oxygen can be achieved only by increasing the ambient pressure above normal. This is a technique which requires a pressure chamber and those in current use raise the ambient pressure from 1 atmosphere (101 kPa) to 2 and for some purposes 3 atmospheres. At 3 atmospheres the plasma content of oxygen is increased to 5.6 ml/dl plasma which is almost sufficient to maintain life without the oxygen linked to haemoglobin, since around 5 ml/dl blood is the basic metabolic requirement.

Toxic effects of oxygen

In patients with respiratory disease depending on 'hypoxic drive' to the respiratory centre to maintain respiration, uncontrolled oxygen administration can lead to *respiratory depression and even apnoea.*

Prolonged oxygen therapy results in *vasoconstriction* and in neonates leads to *retrolental fibroplasia* if concentrations greater than 40 per cent are administered.

Pulmonary damage with oedema may follow prolonged administration of 100 per cent oxygen.

Prolonged exposure to 100 per cent oxygen at increased ambient pressures (2–3 atmospheres) can cause *disturbance to the central nervous system with convulsions.* In addition severe pain in the air sinuses and middle ear may occur.

Methods of administration

There are four main methods of oxygen administration.

Nasal catheter. This method is of use where only a modest increase in the inspired oxygen concentration is desired. Low flows of about

3 litres/minute are well tolerated by the patient and this gives an inspired oxygen concentration of about 25 per cent.

Masks. Many differing types of mask are now available, plastic disposable ones being most popular. Higher flow rates are tolerated by the patient but the flow rate must never be less than the patient's minute volume or rebreathing and carbon dioxide retention will occur. The average adult requires a flow of at least 4 litres of oxygen/minute which will give an inspired oxygen concentration of 50–60 per cent.

Venturi masks. This type of mask, making use of the venturi principle, enables the physician to control more accurately the oxygen concentration administered to the patient. Thus oxygen can be administered to patients with hypoxic drive with less risk of respiratory depression.

The Edinburgh mask (Fig. 10.10). This simple disposable mask is also designed for the delivery of controlled *low concentrations* of oxygen to patients with hypoxic drive.

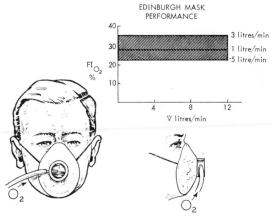

Fig. 10.10 The Edinburgh mask. The inset graph shows the percentage of oxygen in the inspired gas mixture (FI_{O_2}) achieved by delivering different flow rates of oxygen to the open-ended mask. It can be seen that the percentage of oxygen breathed by the patient varies little with changes in the minute volume $\dot{V}$ litres/minute). (After Flenley, D. C., Hutchinson, D. C. S. & Donald, K. W. (1963) *Brit. med. J.* **2,** 1081.)

Oxygen as a vehicle for drug administration
Bronchodilator drugs such as isoprenaline or orciprenaline can be administered in a fine droplet suspension in oxygen using a nebuliser attachment to the administration apparatus. This technique

is useful in patients with bronchospasm particularly when combined with the inhalation of mucolytic agents such as chymotrypsin or 'Alevaire', to liquefy the tenacious sputum. Antiobotics may also be administered in this way although it is more logical and efficient to give them by injection.

Control of oxygen therapy

Quite reasonably, it would be thought rash if a clinician were to administer a potent drug from an uncalibrated syringe. Oxygen is a widely used drug and its safe and effective administration requires similar control. Such control implies measurements of two kinds. First, measurement of the dose administered to the patient and, second, measurement of the effect of the drug on the patient's condition.

Methods of measuring amount of oxygen delivered
Flowmeter. This device measures the flow of oxygen delivered to the patient in litres/minute.

Oxygen analyser. Different types of analyser are available for sampling the inspired concentration (FI_{O_2}) breathed by the patient from mask or ventilator. This measurement should be made at the same time as the patient's arterial oxygen tension is measured in order to relate one to the other.

Methods of assessing therapy
Colour of skin and mucosae. This is unreliable since hypoxaemia can exist in the absence of cyanosis. In addition, lighting conditions and the state of the patient's peripheral circulation can lead to erroneous assessment.

Arterial oxygen measurement. Arterial blood is sampled and the oxygen tension (Pa_{O_2}) estimated. To facilitate repeated measurements in acute illness, indwelling arterial cannulae may be employed.

SEDATIVES, ANALGESICS AND HYPNOTICS

The provision of 'sedation' for patients under his care is one of the first tasks to face the house officer in hospital. By definition, to sedate means *to soothe or settle*, but it is customary to use the term sedative to describe drugs which relieve anxiety, while the terms analgesic and hypnotic are correctly applied to pain-relieving and sleep-producing agents respectively.

There is often an overlap in the actions of a drug, some analgesics, notably the opiates, relieving anxiety and many sedatives, for example the barbiturates, in larger doses inducing sleep. It is therefore essential in selecting the appropriate drug to decide whether the aim is to remedy pain, anxiety or restlessness. It must be remembered also that if a drug is prescribed within a few hours of the beginning or end of an operation it may interact with other drugs used during anaesthesia producing deeper or longer sleep than expected and/or more severe depression of blood pressure or respiration than is desirable. For the safety of the patient, the house officer and the anaesthetist should co-operate in deciding what drugs are to be given immediately before and after operation.

Pain relief

If pain is present an analgesic should be administered. For milder or more chronic pain one may use Tabs. Codein. Co. or Tabs. Paracetamol, one to two, orally, four-hourly. Pain of greater severity may respond to dihydrocodeine bitartrate (DF 118) 30–60 mg or pentazocine 50–75 mg by mouth.

For severe pain, particularly in the post-operative period, the opiates or pethidine are still the drugs of choice. Morphine sulphate 10–15 mg, papaveretum 10–20 mg or pethidine 50–100 mg can be given parenterally for the average adult patient (70 kg body weight). Pentazocine 20–30 mg may be used also. Pentazocine is claimed to be a non-addicting analgesic and is related to the opiate antagonist nalorphine. Its duration of action is shorter than that of morphine but the incidence of emetic sequelae is considerably less. The combination of narcotic analgesics with phenothiazines such as promazine or promethazine increases their sedative effect and reduces the incidence of nausea and vomiting.

The combination of morphine and cyclizine (Cyclimorph) is also worth considering in patients who are experiencing severe pain but have severe nausea and vomiting when opiates are used to relieve the pain. In selecting *the correct dose* consideration should be given to the patient's physical state, his weight and any other drugs given recently. Many anaesthetists give the first post-operative dose of analgesic in dilute solution intravenously, for example morphine 10 mg, or pethidine 100 mg in 10 ml water, taking several minutes to complete the injection and stopping the injection when pain is relieved. This technique is best employed initially under supervision. The opiates provide better psychic sedation than pethidine and in equianalgesic doses (morphine 10 mg = pethidine 60–65 mg) there is little difference in side effects, such as respiratory depression and nausea and vomiting. Papaveretum is claimed to produce less respiratory depression and nausea than does morphine because of the papaverine content but in equi-analgesic dosage with morphine the degree of respiratory and cardiovascular depression is similar. The respiratory depression produced by all three drugs may be antagonised by the intravenous injection of nalorphine 5–10 mg or levallorphan 1–2 mg. Care must be taken not to exceed the dose of these drugs necessary to antagonise the respiratory depression present since this will increase the depression. A new potent narcotic antagonist naloxone (0.1–0.4 mg) may be preferred to nalorphine or levallorphan but like them it not only reverses the depressant effects of the narcotic but also abolishes the analgesia they produce. Narcotic-induced respiratory depression can, however, be reversed without interfering with analgesia by the intravenous administration of a new respiratory stimulant doxapram. This drug is not a true narcotic antagonist but is useful in the post-operative period and is usually administered by continuous intravenous infusion.

NEVER give barbiturates or phenothiazine drugs to a patient suffering from severe pain unless an analgesic is given at the same time. These drugs increase the sensitivity of the patient to pain and cause marked restlessness. Remember also that after operation the peripheral circulation may be impaired and absorption of an opiate injected subcutaneously may be delayed. In these cases, and when using larger or irritant injections, intramuscular injection is indicated.

Relief of anxiety may help to relieve pain and the use of the benzodiazepines is of value. Bear in mind also the value of reassurance and attention to bodily comfort—keeping the patient warm for example. Also of immense value is some form of distraction such as conversation with other patients. Finally, for painful dressings premixed nitrous oxide and oxygen as used in labour (p. 189) may be employed. It may be used also to supplement narcotic therapy preceding and during physiotherapy.

The problem of recognising pain in patients in whom ventilation of the lungs is being controlled mechanically is discussed on page 167.

For the first few days after a major operation an opiate is usually indicated but thereafter night sedation may take the form of a hypnotic along with Tabs. Codein Co. or Tabs. Paracetamol. The change should be made from the more potent drugs as soon as practicable to reduce the liability to addiction.

Anxiety

This occurs commonly in patients in hospital and is all too commonly ignored. Many studies have shown that a patient who approaches surgery in an anxious state requires much more postoperative analgesia. Explanation, reassurance and the administration thrice daily of diazepam 5 mg or other anxiolytic drugs are worthwhile.

Insomnia

There are a vast number of hypnotics from which to choose. Many patients may already have been in the habit of taking such drugs at home and it is often wise to continue the same agent if it has been having a good effect. For the remainder nitrazepam 5–10 mg is considered by many to be the safest hypnotic for long-term use. Of the barbiturates pentobarbitone, quinalbarbitone, butobarbitone or amylobarbitone (100–200 mg orally) all have their advocates. These are best avoided in the elderly lest they cause confusion and glutethimide (Doriden) 250–500 mg or methaqualone 150–300 mg orally are useful alternatives.

Not all hypnotics are equally effective in different individuals and the doctor should be prepared to change if necessary. Many patients may lie awake because of worry which could be largely relieved by daytime anxiolytic therapy.

Restlessness

Restlessness may be associated with pain in the patient recovering from anaesthesia but not yet fully conscious. This restlessness usually responds to an analgesic. In the conscious patient it may be associated with anxiety in which case it responds to a barbiturate or tranquilliser. *Restlessness may be associated with inadequate ventilation or concealed haemorrhage* and these must be excluded as the injudicious use of sedatives may be lethal in such cases. Restlessness may be associated with head injury and may occur in older patients for no obvious reason. Promazine or chlorpromazine 25–50 mg orally or intramuscularly is of value in some of these cases but a specialist opinion is usually desirable before treating a restless patient where the cause is not obvious.

Paraldehyde 10–15 ml orally or rectally, or not more than 0.2 ml/kg intramuscularly should be reserved for otherwise uncontrollable patients.

In conclusion the following are important points to remember:

Always use a drug appropriate to the symptom being treated—analgesics for pain, hypnotics for insomnia, etc.

Learn to use a small number of effective drugs.

Remember the placebo effect. Forty per cent of patients obtain pain relief from injections of saline, and many patients sleep after taking inert tablets. Your drugs must do better than this if they are to be effective.

When dealing with restless patients always look for and deal with the cause if possible. This may involve consulting a senior clinician.

Consider what other drugs the patient has received recently or what other drugs he is likely to receive during anaesthesia or in the post-operative period.

Keep a clear record of all drugs given, their dosage, route, time of administration and effect, where others will see the record before further drugs are prescribed.

Do not prescribe powerful drugs to be given 'four- or six-hourly' as a routine. Many are cumulative, and the need for further injection should be established.

11

The respiratory intensive care unit

The post-operative recovery phase usually lasts from 1 to 24 hours. However, certain patients may require much longer special care and they are best accommodated in an intensive care unit, where other patients, not necessarily in the post-operative period, are nursed intensively for longer periods of time, for example two days to six weeks.

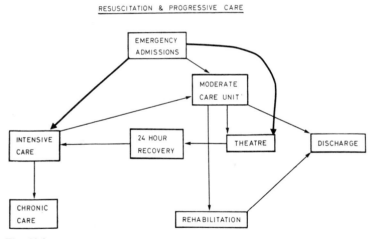

RESUSCITATION & PROGRESSIVE CARE

Fig. 11.1

This pattern of progressive care of patients throughout their stay in hospital can be applied more widely than to surgical patients alone. Figure 11.1 shows the various pathways the patient may follow after reception at an emergency admission unit until his ultimate discharge from hospital. In any individual case the sole consideration which determines the patient's place of treatment is the degree of observation and the amount of therapy required. The most ill patients, therefore, are gathered together in areas where staff and equipment are concentrated to enable intensive observation and therapy to be undertaken. Intensive care areas are made up of individual units restricted to the treatment of a particular group of patients such as those with respiratory or renal failure and myocardial infarction.

The anaesthetist is concerned mainly with that part of the intensive care area where patients with respiratory problems are treated, and it is this type of patient whom we shall consider here. The following are some of the conditions which can lead to a patient's admission to the respiratory intensive care unit.

Post-operative respiratory insufficiency.

Severe head injuries and facio-maxillary injuries.

Trauma to the chest wall: crushed-chest injuries.

Obstructive lung disease with respiratory failure (emphysema with an additional acute respiratory infection).

Carbon monoxide and barbiturate poisoning.

Certain infectious diseases: poliomyelitis, polyneuritis, tetanus.

Miscellaneous medical conditions: cerebrovascular accidents, myasthenia gravis, acute porphyria.

A proportion of patients admitted to the intensive care unit will require general supportive therapy while under close and continuous observation. The majority, however, will require more vigorous treatment aimed at augmenting inadequate respiratory effort and specific therapy.

SPECIAL PROCEDURES IN THE RESPIRATORY UNIT

The methods and manœuvres used in the recovery room are, of course, also practised in the respiratory unit, but a knowledge of some additional procedures is essential.

Parenteral feeding
Particular attention should be paid to the nutritional requirements of all patients in the intensive care unit. So far as post-trauma and post-operative patients are concerned, it is very common for a metabolic or nutritional problem to be revealed as a major factor in their illness although all these patients have been admitted primarily as respiratory problems.

The two commoner potential causes of starvation in these patients are excessive catabolism, or breakdown of tissue, following injury or major surgery and malabsorption from the gastrointestinal tract where there is some degree of paralytic ileus. Both factors may be present and be aggravated further by the presence of sepsis. A fully balanced diet of adequate calorific content and containing sufficient protein should be given by mouth wherever possible to suit the individual requirements. If the patient cannot swallow, the diet can be liquefied and given via a nasogastric tube. If this is not attainable within a few hours of admission then full intravenous feeding is instituted. Solutions of essential amino-acids are available, the building materials from which tissue proteins are constructed in the body, and also solutions of intravenous fats and concentrated sugars, to provide the calorific energy required for metabolism in general and tissue repair in particular.

Table 11.1 Intravenous diet for a 24-hour period in a 70 kg adult

Solution	Volume ml	Calories	Nitrogen content (grams/litre)
Amino-acids (e.g. Trophysan conc. 10%)	1000	724	12.8
Fat emulsion (e.g. Lipiphysan 10%)	500	620	0
Carbohydrate (e.g. Sorbital 30%)	1500	1800	0
Total	3000	3144	12.8

NOTE: The fat and amino-acid solutions are usually given simultaneously with the sugar solution using a 'Y' drip. One bottle of carbohydrate (500 ml) can be replaced by a bottle of normal saline or other electrolyte solution if required. Other electrolyte supplements, e.g. potassium, are given as required, as are vitamin supplements.

Table 11.2 Intravenous diet for a 24-hour period in a 20 kg child

Solution	Volume ml	Calories	Nitrogen content (grams/litre)
Amino-acids (e.g. Trophysan 5%)	500	182	6.68
Fat emulsion (e.g. Lipiphysan 10%)	250	310	0
Carbohydrate (e.g. Sorbitol 30%)	250	300	0
Total	1000	792	7

NOTE: Additional fluid requirements can be met by adding dextrose/water or half-strength normal saline in appropriate volume. Vitamin and electrolyte supplements must also be added.

These solutions are hypertonic and are therefore best given via a large vein, usually the superior or inferior vena cava. If peripheral veins are used the site of infusion must frequently be changed to avoid thrombophlebitis developing.

Particular care is required when administering intravenous fat emulsions since some patients may produce an allergic type reaction requiring the discontinuing of the infusion and the administration of an antihistamine such as chlorpheniramine maleate (Piriton). Fat emulsions are also contra-indicated in pregnancy, liver disease and where there is a blood disease with an increased bleeding tendency. Nevertheless, the ability to provide full nutritional requirements parenterally is a most valuable therapeutic measure in the intensive care of these severely ill patients. Two diets are listed above, one suitable for an adult and one for a child requiring intravenous feeding.

Tracheostomy

If assistance to ventilation is required it is usually necessary to insert a cuffed endotracheal tube (see p. 101). This enables secretions in the bronchi to be aspirated and usually ensures an unobstructed airway. The tracheal tube is a temporary expedient and is not commonly left in place beyond 24–48 hours. For longer periods of treatment an uncuffed nasotracheal tube may be used particularly in children. Where this type of assistance is required for an indefinite period it is usual to perform a tracheostomy.

Indications

Although the operation is performed for many varying surgical and medical conditions these fall readily into two main groups:

1. Conditions in which there is *obstruction to the patient's airway*, particularly in its upper part, for example acute oedema of the glottis and carcinoma of larynx. The value of tracheostomy is obvious here—the obstruction is bypassed and free and tranquil breathing ensues.
2. Conditions in which *impairment of the patient's respiratory function*, other than simple airway obstruction, is a threat to life. The causes of respiratory insufficiency have been dealt with already (Chap. 9) and may vary from acute trauma to poliomyelitis. Usually such patients have no cough or, at best, an ineffective one and secretions accumulate rapidly in the airway and must be removed.

Advantages of tracheostomy
— Some *reduction of the physiological dead-space* formed by the upper air passages results. This may marginally improve alveolar ventilation.
— Easier *removal of secretions* from the air passages.
—A *reduction in the work of ventilation* and in oxygen requirements results from 1 and 2.
— *Better control of oxygen administration* is possible via a tracheostomy box and humidifier (Fig. 11.2).

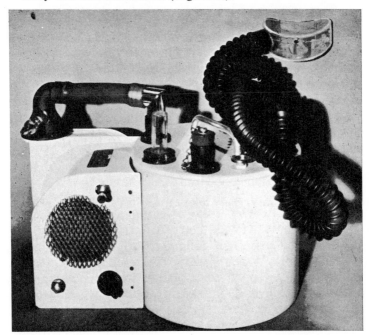

Fig. 11.2 The perspex tracheostomy box is shown in the right upper portion of the photograph, in this case connected by the corrugated tubing to a humidifier.

— In patients with depressed cough and swallowing reflexes, the lungs can be *sealed off from the danger of aspirated secretions and gastric contents*, by the use of a cuffed tracheostomy tube (Fig. 11.3).
— Should *mechanical assistance to ventilation* be required in addition, this is facilitated by a tracheostomy.

Management of tracheostomy
In order that the patient may benefit fully from this procedure certain problems of management must be understood and overcome.

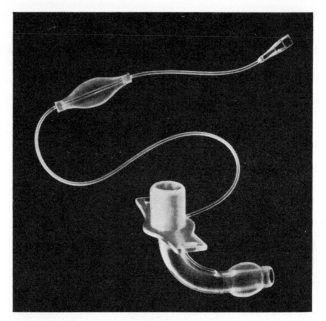

Fig. 11.3 The Portex disposable tracheostomy tube.

Care of tubes. It is customary to insert a tube through the tracheostomy opening into the trachea. The familiar double-silver tube is still used, but usually when the patient is on the way to recovery. In the early stages, however, one of the cuffed variety is preferred, as this type of tube provides an effective seal for the lungs against secretions and makes possible assisted or controlled ventilation, should this be required. Over-inflation of the cuff for long periods can lead to excessive pressure on the tracheal mucosa and to necrosis and sloughing. This can be avoided by inflation of the cuff to make a seal without excessive pressure and, by deflation of the cuff at intervals, for a short time. Deflation of the cuff must always be preceded by thorough oropharyngeal suction so that secretions will not run down alongside the tube into the lungs. To reduce these hazards further new tubes have been introduced including double-cuffed ones, where each cuff is inflated alternately for a period, and also low-pressure single-cuffed tubes, where there is less pressure applied to the tracheal mucosa. Tubes must be changed frequently, particularly when the sputum is copious and viscid, since the inside becomes encrusted with dried secretions. Otherwise the lumen of the tube gradually becomes blocked and death from acute asphyxia may result. Tracheostomy tubes are usually changed at least every 48 hours.

Humidification. Since the paranasal sinuses and nasopharynx, whose function is to warm and humidify the inspired air, have been bypassed by the tracheostomy, it is necessary to provide an alternative source of moisture and heat, to avoid hardening of the secretions and drying and fissuring of the mucosa of the respiratory tract. This can be done in various ways:

— It may be sufficient to inject small quantities (0.5 ml) of sterile saline down the tracheostomy tube at intervals.
— If the patient is breathing room air, then, in a humid climate, it is often sufficient to conserve the moisture in the patient's own expirations with a simple condenser humidifier (Fig. 11.4).

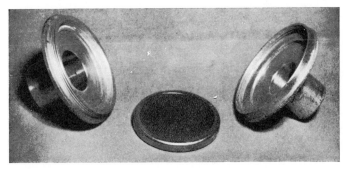

Fig. 11.4 The condenser humidifier: The two parts of the humidifier have been unscrewed to reveal the removable wire-gauze insert.

The moisture in each expiration condenses on the wire-mesh and revaporises on inspiration. Condenser humidifiers are efficient only when the mesh remains reasonably dry and so it must be changed repeatedly, usually three-hourly, and dried. The wire-mesh serves also to trap large dust particles and prevent their inhalation.

— In a dry climate, where the atmosphere contains little water vapour, or when the patient breathes oxygen, which is delivered free of moisture and fairly cold from the cylinder or pipe-line, active warming and humidification is usually required. This is done by passing the oxygen or air/oxygen mixture through a 'tank' type humidifier (Fig. 11.5) which warms the gas to about body temperature and saturates it with water vapour. The warm and moist oxygen then passes along a tube to a perspex tracheostomy box (Fig. 11.2) mounted over the tracheostomy tube. This box has a series of holes in its surface to permit free expiration and elimination of carbon dioxide

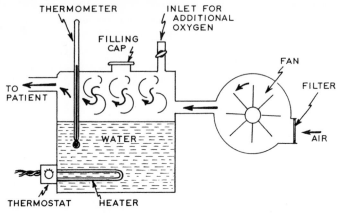

Fig. 11.5 The tank humidifier: Air or air and oxygen or blown over the surface of the warm water and then to the patient.

which would otherwise accumulate. There is also a port-hole, with a cover which slides to one side, to give access for tracheal suction. An alternative to the tracheostomy box is a plastic 'T' piece mounted on the tracheostomy tube (Fig. 11.6).
— Other devices designed to solve the problem of humidification act like perfume 'atomisers' and propel a fine spray of water droplets into the stream of air or oxygen as it is inspired. These devices have the advantage that bronchodilator drugs, such as isoprenaline (Neo-Epinine), salbutamol (Ventolin), or anti-biotics, may be suspended in the water and delivered into the depths of the lungs.

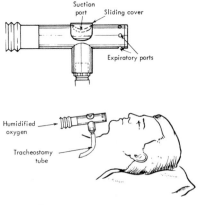

Fig. 11.6 A tracheostomy T piece.

Before leaving the subject of humidification it is necessary to mention, if only to condemn, the practice of 'humidifying' oxygen by bubbling it through a Wolff's bottle. This device is not an efficient method of adding moisture to the inspired gases.

Endobronchial suction. The care with which secretions are aspirated from the patient's airway is of the greatest importance. The accent should always be on sterility, thoroughness and gentleness.

It is obvious that the patient is at risk from whatever lethal organism is carelessly introduced because of inadequate sterile technique. If not of the disposable type the endobronchial catheters should be used only once and then cleaned and autoclaved. The catheter used for oropharyngeal suction should not be used for suction through the tracheostomy. The hands should be scrubbed before each period of suction and should never come in contact with that portion of the catheter which enters the patient's airway.

Tracheal suction should be carried out as often as is necessary to keep the airways free from secretions. The more copious the secretions, the more often must the manœuvre be repeated. Whenever possible two people should co-operate during this time, one carrying out the aspiration and the other turning the patient from one side to the other to ensure that the catheter enters both right and left main bronchi.

The calibre of the catheter selected is important. Its diameter should be less than half that of the tracheostomy tube, otherwise it will block it partially or completely and cause acute asphyxia. The catheter should be occluded between finger and thumb when introduced and released to allow suction only on withdrawal, otherwise there is a danger that excessive suction will collapse portions of the lung. The negative pressure should never be greater than is required to remove the secretions easily. More powerful suction is required when the sputum is thick and tenacious. At all times, the catheter should be handled gently to avoid unnecessary trauma to the sensitive mucosa of the respiratory tract.

Complications of tracheostomy
Infection. Tracheostomy opens up a route for secondary infection of the lungs and hence the management of such cases must be attended by scrupulous aseptic precautions.

Loss of humidification. Loss of the normal humidification of the inspired gases by the paranasal sinuses and nasopharynx results in crusting of secretions in the airway.

Mucosal ulceration. As a result of excessive pressure in the tracheostomy tube cuff.

Dilatation of the trachea. Over-inflation of the tube cuff may result in erosion of the cartilaginous rings of the trachea and resultant dilatation.

Granuloma. Trauma to the tracheal mucosa may cause the development of granulation tissue and a small polyp may result.

Fistula formation. This is a serious complication which may occur rarely. Excessive cuff pressure and other trauma lead to the formation of a tracheo-oesophageal fistula. Food and secretions enter the trachea below the cuff of the tube and contaminate the lungs.

Sinus formation. Imperfect healing of the post-tracheostomy stoma can result in a persistent sinus requiring surgical closure.

Erosion of blood vessels. Particularly if the stoma becomes infected, a blood vessel may be eroded by the tracheostomy tube, causing severe haemorrhage.

Tracheal stricture. In about 2 per cent of patients with a tracheostomy, who have had ventilator treatment, a stricture may develop either at the site of the cuff or at the lower end of the tube. This is a serious late complication often requiring difficult plastic surgery. It is commoner in young children where the cross-section of the airway is quite small. Nasotracheal intubation is preferred to tracheostomy in children to avoid this.

Mechanical assistance to ventilation (intermittent positive pressure ventilation: IPPV)

There are two main groups of patients outside of the operating theatre who require mechanical assistance to ventilation:

Those with *demonstrable respiratory failure* from whatever cause. This may be defined, from the point of view of blood chemistry, as being present where the arterial oxygen tension is less than 50 mmHg (6.7 kPa) or where the arterial carbon dioxide tension exceeds 50 mmHg.

Those patients in whom *respiratory failure may be confidently anticipated*. Examples of this group are to be seen where patients with gross cardiopulmonary disease are to undergo emergency surgery, in extremely obese patients in the post-operative period and patients with gross metabolic disturbance.

Before embarking on a description of mechanical assistance to ventilation it is necessary to consider some physiological aspects of the technique (Fig. 11.7). Controlled ventilation, whether performed manually or mechanically, has certain potentially harmful effects on the respiratory and cardiovascular systems. Excessive pressures applied to the patient's airway may result in damage to lung tissue and even to rupture of the lungs. It is generally accepted that pressures exceeding $+30$ cm H_2O at the mouth should be avoided and most machines in use incorporate a safety

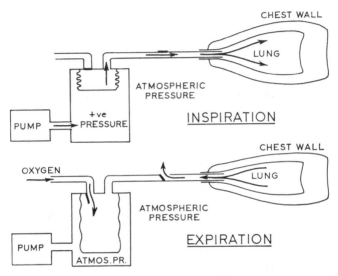

Fig. 11.7 Diagram of ventilator action: The bellows or bag containing the fresh gases is enclosed in an airtight chamber and squeezed during inspiration by the action of a pump which raises the pressure inside the chamber above the outside or atmospheric pressure. Thus the fresh gases are propelled into the patient's lungs through the endotracheal tube. During expiration, the pressure in the chamber falls again to atmospheric and the expired gases flow out of the lungs, escaping to the outside air through a valve. At the same time, the bellows fill with fresh gas in readiness for the next inspiration.

valve which opens automatically when the airway pressure exceeds this figure. In addition a pressure gauge is attached to the ventilator which gives a continuous reading of the pressure at the ventilator outlet and in some cases at the attachment to the patient's airway. The volume of gases entering or leaving the lungs is recorded on a spirometer or is pre-set by adjusting a control on the machine. Thus continuous observations of the tidal volume and cycling pressure of the ventilator and the frequency of ventilation can be made by the anaesthetist. The patient's ventilation requirements are predicted before operation ·from such factors as body weight, sex, etc., and the ventilator can be adjusted to meet these requirements. Where there is doubt remaining, blood-gas analysis, or analysis of the expired gas in the case of carbon dioxide, can be carried out at intervals to ensure adequate oxygenation and adequate elimination of carbon dioxide.

The potentially harmful effects of intermittent positive pressure ventilation on the cardiovascular system can result in a reduction in cardiac output and lead to cardiac failure. The explanation of this is to be found when we compare the intrathoracic pressure changes which accompany spontaneous respiration with those occurring during controlled ventilation. Normally the intrapulmonary and intrapleural pressures are negative during inspiration and this assists the venous return to the right side of the heart—the 'thoracic pump' mechanism. During expiration, the intrapulmonary pressure is positive and the intrapleural pressure is still negative although reduced. When controlled ventilation is undertaken the mean intrapleural pressure is less negative and may become positive. Therefore, there is some interference with central venous return and obstruction to the pulmonary blood flow. The normal individual is able to compensate for these effects, but in severely ill or shocked patients there may be a reduction in cardiac output and hypotension.

The use of a negative phase during the expiratory cycle of the ventilator will minimise this cardiovascular disturbance. This negative pressure should not exceed -5 cm H_2O or it may lead to collapse of diseased bronchioles in patients with chronic respiratory disease. Other patterns of mechanical ventilation can be used in selected patients. For instance, where pulmonary oedema is a problem or where there is likely to be premature closure of the smaller bronchioles during the expiratory cycle, a positive pressure of 5 to 10 cm H_2O may be applied towards the end of this cycle of the machine. This is known as *positive end expiratory pressure* (PEEP), but it must be used with great care since the effect may be to embarrass further the cardiac output. Some patients may be difficult to 'wean' from the machine following a period of ventilator therapy, and this stage in treatment can be facilitated by arranging to augment the patient's own inadequate respiratory efforts in various ways. One method employs a 'trigger' set to change the action of the machine automatically to follow any spontaneous efforts the patient may make (patient-assisted or triggered ventilation). Another technique permits the patient to breathe spontaneously through an alternative circuit but the ventilator provides a regular boost to the patient's own breathing at a pre-set rate and tidal volume. This is called *intermittent mandatory ventilation* (IMV).

The manual method of ventilation, using a device such as the Ambu resuscitator (Fig. 10.2) is convenient in emergencies and for short periods of time.

Management of patient's undergoing artificial ventilation
Successful management of patients undergoing artificial ventilation requires the highest standards of skill and care. Figure 11.8 summarises some of the most important aspects of this treatment.

Routine tracheostomy regime
The routine care as for other tracheostomy cases is carried out but with one important modification. Most of the patients on ventilators are not breathing at all and can therefore only be disconnected for very short periods (approximately one minute) at a time to permit endobronchial suction. It is usually necessary to perform each period of suction in stages, allowing the patient a few breaths on the machine between each stage.

The management of pain
During ventilator therapy the provision of adequate pain relief can present difficulties, especially in the patient who is unable to communicate. Although the available drugs and techniques of pain relief are many and varied, they are of little value in a situation where the clinician is unable to detect a need for them.

The patient normally reacts to unmodified pain in three ways:

by making avoidance movements: attempting to withdraw the injured portion of the body from the stimulus

by responding autonomically: by changes in heart rate and systolic blood pressure

by responding at a cortical level in perceiving the 'painful' stimulus and evaluating it against previous similar experience

Many of the patients undergoing artificial ventilation are incapable of the first response and indeed may be curarised. Although it has been claimed that the clinician can detect the higher response by complicated electroencephalographic techniques, this is impractical clinically. Measurements of the autonomic response are as yet the only practicable approach in this difficult situation.

The important thing for the clinician to remember is that an immobile, apparently tranquil, patient may be suffering from

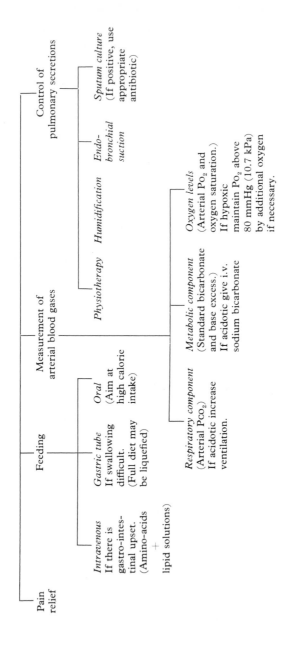

Fig. 11.8 Management of patient during artificial ventilation.

considerable pain and its relief is an urgent matter. The method and drugs chosen will vary with the individual circumstances but the following list indicates the possibilities:

Parenteral analgesia. Generally speaking, the intravenous route is to be preferred in this situation since the timing of the peak effect can be more certain and also the relief of pain achieved more quickly. Small incremental doses of 2 mg morphine sulphate, for example, are given intravenously until relief is obtained.

Inhalation analgesia. It is technically simple with apparatus now available to administer inhalation agents to the patient receiving ventilator therapy, although this method is seldom employed to provide pain relief. A 50 per cent mixture of nitrous oxide in oxygen (Entonox: BOC) is probably the best of the available anaesthetic agents which could be given in this way.

Regional blockade. Where it is possible to induce a regional block, complete analgesia of the affected part without any risk of central depression can be achieved. The treatment can be repeated at intervals or maintained continuously as in the case of an epidural block.

General care and physiotherapy

These patients must receive particular attention to pressure areas, oral hygiene, eyes and nose. The use of a 'ripple-mattress' greatly reduces the chance of bed-sores developing. Many will have in-dwelling urinary catheters on continuous drainage and in-travenous infusions which need constant attention. Passive main-tenance exercises to the limbs, percussion of the chest wall and postural drainage are carried out regularly and the physiotherapist has an important function in the treatment of these patients.

Nutrition

When a patient's illness is not severe or is of short duration, in-adequate nutrition may not lead to serious consequences. In trau-matised patients who are receiving an inadequate calorie intake, the amount of tissue protein breakdown and nitrogen lost may be two to three times that in straightforward starvation. For every 10 g of nitrogen excreted in the urine approximately 300 g of muscle protein is lost and this process of catabolism is roughly proportional to the severity of surgery or trauma and is aggravated by the presence of sepsis. The patient in an intensive care unit who is gravely ill and in whom sepsis and abnormal electrolyte loss is present requires the most careful dietary care if a protracted stay in the unit or indeed a fatal outcome is to be avoided. In the past the metabolic response to severe illness or gross trauma was thought to be unavoidable. It is now known that the negative nitrogen balance which is a feature in these patients is largely reversible if food over and above the patient's normal requirement is provided.

The route of choice is by mouth if the patient is able to swallow and if there is no gastro-intestinal upset. If the patient cannot swallow then the patient can be tube fed. Where there is a gastro-intestinal upset such as paralytic ileus following surgery or injury it is possible to provide an adequate dietary intake intravenously employing amino-acid solutions along with concentrated sugar solutions or fat emulsions as a source of calories. As the patient recovers, feeding by way of a nasal gastric tube will take the place of the intravenous infusions. The feeds are given in small bulk of high calorie value and with additional vitamin supplements. When the patient is able to swallow satisfactorily, oral feeding with a soft liquid diet is instituted. The dietitian's advice on nutritional problems can be invaluable at this stage and hasten the recovery process.

Recording of vital functions
In addition to the regular recording of arterial pressure, central venous pressure (Fig. 11.9), heart rate and temperature, it is important that the nurse, under the direction of the anaesthetist,

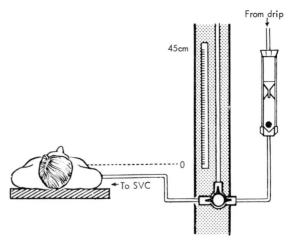

Fig. 11.9 A central venous pressure manometer system. The zero point on the scale is levelled with the right atrium.

Time and Date	O_2 Sat. or P_{O_2}	pH	P_{CO_2}	Stand Bicarb.	Base Excess	Buffer Base	On Ventilator			Off Ventilator			Air Entry in Lungs		Remarks
							f	V_T	P	f	V_T		Left	Right	

Fig. 11.10 Ventilation Chart: key to symbols

O_2 saturation (O_2 sat.): the percentage of haemoglobin saturated with oxygen in the arterial blood.
P_{O_2}: tension of oxygen in arterial blood.
pH: the degree of acidity or alkalinity of the blood in pH units.
P_{CO_2}: the tension of carbon dioxide in the arterial blood. This is high in respiratory failure.

Standard bicarbonate ⎫
Base excess   ⎬ These measurements indicate the efficiency of ventilation and the body metabolism.
Buffer base   ⎭

f: respiratory rate.
V_T: tidal volume.
P: the ventilator pressure during ventilation.
Air entry into lungs: A + or − in this column indicates the nurse's assessment of the degree of lung inflation using a stethoscope.

should observe closely and record certain aspects of the ventilator's performance during treatment (Fig. 11.10). For each patient under treatment an ideal pattern of ventilation will have been chosen with regard to frequency of respiration, airway pressure (that is, the pressure at the patient's mouth during each respiratory cycle of the machine) and the volume of gas being delivered to the patient's lungs (Fig. 11.11). Most respiratory units have a chart on which these events, together with other relevant data, are recorded. The nurse is also trained to listen with a stethoscope

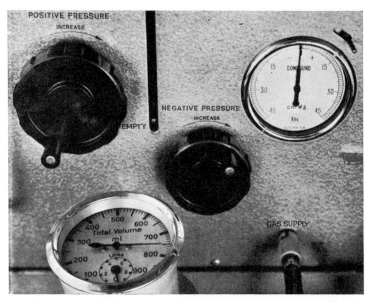

Fig. 11.11 The Dräger respirometer attached to a ventilator can be seen in the left lower corner of the illustration. The gauge on the right measures the pressure required to inflate the patient's lungs.

over both lungs, at intervals, to make sure that the gases are entering the lungs and not being prevented from doing so by secretions in the upper airway or an obstructed tracheostomy tube.

During the intervals when the patient is disconnected from the ventilator to assess his ability to breathe spontaneously the nurse may be asked to make measurements of the tidal volume as well as the frequency of respiration. For this purpose a spirometer such as the Wright's model can be employed (Fig. 5.3).

Information about the patient's arterial blood-gas levels (oxygen saturation, Po_2, pH, Pco_2 and base excess), during intermittent positive pressure ventilation, is usually recorded on the ventilation chart by the anaesthetist and the pattern of ventilation may have to be changed at intervals to keep these levels as near normal as possible. The maintenance of electrolyte and water balance can be difficult in such cases and it is of the first importance to keep *accurate* records on a suitable *Input–Output* Chart. The hourly measurement of urine volume may be necessary in the most severely ill, and renal function may be assessed further by regular measurement of urine and plasma osmolality.

Monitoring.

In order to permit frequent, accurate measurements to be made in the most gravely ill patients, many vital functions are continuously measured and displayed electrically or even automatically charted at predetermined intervals. Alarm systems can also be incorporated to warn when heart rate or arterial pressure, etc., change beyond pre-set limits (see Fig. 11.12).

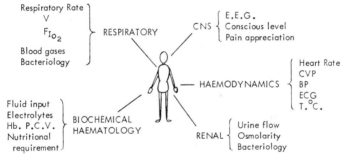

Fig. 11.12 Schematic diagram demonstrating the wide range of measurements required to guide the clinician in the management of a gravely ill patient in an intensive care unit.

The control of infection

The operation of tracheostomy has been described as potentially lethal in that it opens up a direct route for infection to enter the patient's lungs. In addition, all the patients in an intensive care unit are severely ill and prone to intercurrent infection and it is therefore of the utmost importance to minimise the risk of cross-infection from one patient to the other and to isolate any cases of known infection by barrier nursing. Bed-stations should be at least 12 to 14 feet apart since this measure alone greatly reduces the risk of cross-infection. To facilitate isolation of infected cases cubicles are essential, preferably with separate entrances and exits.

A further measure which is of considerable assistance is to ventilate intensive care units, in the same manner as operating theatres, with filtered air from a positive pressure plenum system. Additional filters can be fitted to suction pumps and ventilator air-pumps to further safeguard the patients. All staff working in the unit should observe the accepted rules governing dress and conduct pertaining in operating theatres.

Staff–patient relationships
Many patients undergoing artificial ventilation are fully conscious but because of the tracheostomy cannot make their wants known to the nurse or doctor in the usual way. Often they become acutely distressed and despite continuing physical improvement lose their will to fight. The presence of understanding and cheerful staff can go a long way towards mitigating what is, for most, a strange and terrifying experience. Some may be able to write their requests and should always have a pad of paper and pencil at hand, but for others it is necessary to provide a large alphabet on which the patient can spell out a message with a finger. Great patience is required at this stage and one must be prepared to spend a lot of time in keeping up the patient's morale.

THE UNCONSCIOUS PATIENT

A varying proportion of the patients in the respiratory intensive care area are unconscious. Some of these may have head injuries alone or along with other injuries. Recording the level of unconsciousness is important and may be difficult. Accurate observations recorded frequently can be invaluable in assessing whether improvement or deterioration is taking place. This vitally important task of monitoring these patients can be much assisted if a standard method of recording any changes is adopted. One such chart, developed in the Institute of Neurological Sciences at Glasgow, is illustrated in Figure 11.13. The nurse regularly charts the 'best response' so far as eye-opening, speech and motor activity are concerned at regular intervals, and the clinician can see at a glance how the patient's neurological status is changing, if at all.

Other observations helpful in assessing these patients are rate, depth and character of respiration, rate and volume of pulse, arterial pressure and central venous pressure. In certain neurosurgical cases intracranial pressure changes can be measured directly by means of a cannula inserted through a burr-hole in the skull into the ventricle but this, of course, carries an added risk of introducing infection.

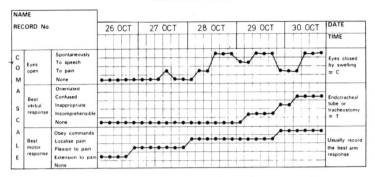

Fig. 11.13 The Glasgow coma scale showing observations on a patient over a 5-day period.

ACUTE POISONING

Death from poisoning now rivals that from road accidents in this country. About two-thirds of these deaths are non-accidental with the number of females exceeding that of males. Accidental deaths from poisoning are almost exclusively confined to children under 10 years of age.

Of those patients who reach hospital alive, some 10 per cent require the full facilities of an intensive care unit if they are to survive. Following the initial resuscitation and gastric lavage where indicated, the most important aspect of treatment is to maintain a clear airway and support respiration if this is depressed. General supportive measures may also be directed to support depressed cardiovascular function and in some patients to rewarm from a hypothermic state. The techniques already described are therefore applicable in these gravely ill patients and if applied vigorously are usually sufficient to ensure ultimate recovery. In certain instances, however, additional treatment is also aimed at increasing the rate of elimination of the ingested poison from the body and it is appropriate to outline these techniques here, since in many hospitals they are used in the respiratory intensive care unit as well as the renal unit.

Forced diuresis
Forced diuresis is the most commonly employed method to increase the rate of excretion of a drug from the body. It is of most value when a long-acting barbiturate such as sodium phenobarbitone has been taken by the patient. Briefly the aim is to increase

the urine flow so as to 'wash-out' the drug and this process is made more efficient if the urine is kept alkaline. Since it is possible to overload the patient with fluids given in large quantities intravenously it is wise to make regular measurements of central venous pressure during treatment in addition to auscultating the lungs for signs of pulmonary oedema.

A suitable regime for forced diuresis is as follows:

Establish closed urinary drainage. This is an essential preliminary to facilitate the measurement of urine flow at hourly intervals.
Establish an intravenous infusion. This is best done by setting up a caval cannula as for central venous pressure measurement. These measurements should be made regularly during the forced diuresis. The infusion is normally begun with 1 litre of normal saline in the first hour followed by 500 ml of 5 per cent dextrose solution in the second hour.

An intravenous diuretic such as frusemide (Lasix) is given (20–80 mg) in repeated doses to maintain a satisfactory urine flow. The fluid input should not be allowed to exceed the output by more than 1 litre and indeed less if there is any sign of circulatory embarrassment.

If the diuresis is adequate then the intravenous infusion is continued in the following way.

1. 500 ml 5 per cent dextrose in water plus 50 mmol sodium bicarbonate.
2. 500 ml 5 per cent dextrose in water plus 24 mmol potassium chloride.
3. 500 ml normal saline.

Those three solutions are rotated and given at the rate of 500 ml per hour for the duration of treatment. The sodium bicarbonate is given to maintain an alkaline state and the potassium supplement to replace potassium lost in the urine during the diuresis.

Peritoneal dialysis
This technique is occasionally employed as an adjunct to forced diuresis or where haemodialysis is impracticable. Under aseptic conditions a catheter is inserted below the umbilicus under local analgesia. The peritoneal cavity is then lavaged with a dialysing solution containing antibiotic. Figure 11.14 shows the arrangement of the apparatus attached to the catheter. The aim is to use the peritoneum as a dialysing membrane and thus expedite

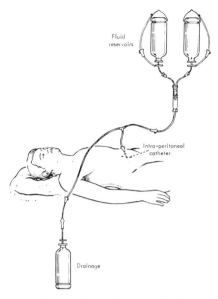

Fluid
reservoirs

Intra-peritoneal
catheter

Drainage

Fig. 11.14 Apparatus in use during peritoneal dialysis.

removal of the ingested drug from the body. Usually one litre of solution is run in over about 20 minutes. The solution is then allowed to remain for about 20 minutes before being drained off. This cycle is repeated hourly for the duration of treatment.

Haemodialysis
The most severely poisoned patients may require haemodialysis. Here the patient's blood is circulated through an artificial kidney machine, some of the drug removed from the blood and the blood returned to the patient.

Haemoperfusion
Recently, this new technique has been introduced into clinical practice. The patient's blood is circulated extracorporeally through a container of activated charcoal which adsorbs the drug. The apparatus is cheap, compact and effective.

It cannot be emphasised too strongly that, while these methods may assist the patient's recovery, survival depends on vigorous application of the general supportive measures already described, in particular those directed towards the support of respiratory function.

12

Resuscitation

EXPIRED AIR RESUSCITATION OR MOUTH-TO-MOUTH BREATHING

History

Probably the first written account of this ancient technique is to be found in the Old Testament in the Second Book of Kings. There, a description is given of the resuscitation of a young boy by the prophet Elisha and for many hundreds of years the method was known as Elisha breathing. In 1954 Elam and his colleagues demonstrated that expired air resuscitation was more effective than the standard methods of artificial respiration, for example Holger–Nielson and Schafer methods. In 1958 Safar described an airway he designed to make the method easier to perform and in 1960 the Brook airway was first produced.

Table 12.1 Constituents of air samples (approximate values)

Gas	Atmospheric air %	Alveolar air %	Expired air %
Oxygen	21	14.5	14–18
Carbon dioxide	0.04	5.5	4.5
Nitrogen and water vapour	79	80	79

It will be noted from Table 12.1 that atmospheric air contains about 21 per cent oxygen and minimal carbon dioxide. Provided an adequate amount of air is propelled into the depths of the lungs by the bellows action of the chest and diaphragm, and the airway is clear, the blood flowing through the pulmonary capillaries will be sufficiently oxygenated (the haemoglobin will be at least 95 per cent saturated with oxygen). In addition, the carbon dioxide carried to the lungs from the tissues will be effectively removed and vented to the atmosphere.

This process of normal ventilation can, of course, be replaced fairly effectively in patients with respiratory arrest by using a belows like the Ambu resuscitator to ventilate the lungs with air (atmospheric air resuscitation). Provided the operator compresses the bellows often enough, the tidal volume is adequate, and the airway is clear, the patient will come to no harm.

It is less easy to understand how the expired air of the 'donor' is adequate to resuscitate a patient. From Table 12.1 it can be seen that expired air contains 14–18 per cent oxygen and 4.5 per cent carbon dioxide. Thus there is more oxygen and less carbon dioxide than in alveolar air; the latter is mixed with the unused atmospheric air in the air passages on expiration (dead-space air). Expired air has been shown to be sufficient to maintain life in volunteers whose respiratory muscles have been temporarily paralysed with curare. In this instance, the victim's arterial blood will contain an adequate quantity of oxygen (the haemoglobin will be about 80 per cent saturated with oxygen) and the carbon dioxide level will remain sufficiently low over long periods of time, for example 40 minutes.

During expired air resuscitation the donor uses his lungs and diaphragm to inflate the victim's lungs. In this way an adequate tidal volume can be maintained.

Technique

This is best learned on one of the model patients now available, for example the Ambu manikin or 'Resuscianne'. All medical and nursing personnel should receive a course of instruction and demonstration and should practise the method for themselves. The correct use of the Safar and Brook airways (Fig. 12.1) which facilitate the technique can be learned at the same time and also the use of the bellows resuscitator for atmospheric air resuscitation (Fig. 12.2).

The following points must be observed:

— Place the victim on his back if possible.
— Secure a clear airway by posturing the head, removing mucus from the mouth and supporting the lower jaw with the hand to keep the tongue forward (Fig. 9.2).
— Apply your mouth to the victim's, making a good seal to prevent leakage of air. In the adult, the nostrils must also be pinched with the fingers of the left hand. In the child, the donor's mouth covers the victim's nostrils and mouth.
— Blow until you see the chest rise, removing your mouth to permit expiration. If the stomach fills with air then gentle pressure over it will empty it. The head must then be correctly

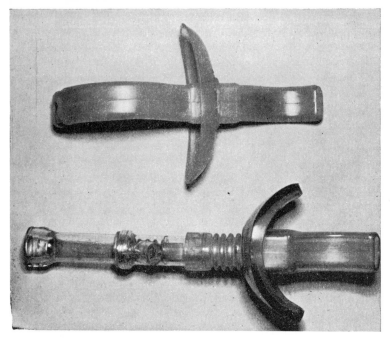

Fig. 12.1 The Safar airway (above) and the Brook airway (below).

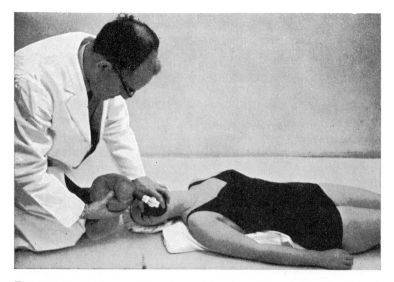

Fig. 12.2 The Ambu resuscitator in use. Note the position of the patient's head.

postured to improve the airway and prevent a recurrence. If regurgitation of stomach contents takes place the airway must be again cleared before continuing with the resuscitation.

— Repeat the inflation of the chest 10–20 times/minute.
— Continue until the patient is breathing adequately for himself or further help and equipment arrive.
— If the jaw muscles are in spasm and the mouth cannot be opened then the 'mouth-to-nose' route may be employed after the usual posturing of the head. The latter technique is, in fact, preferred by some experts in all cases.

Advantages and disadvantages

There is only *one* apparent *disadvantage* and that is the natural reluctance of the donor to carry out a manœuvre requiring such intimate contact with the victim. The risk of infection is minimal but in any case such a risk must be weighed against the reward of a successful resuscitation.

Advantages of mouth-to-mouth breathing

The *advantages* of the method are self-evident.

— No complicated apparatus is required.
— The technique is easy to learn and superior to all other methods of artificial respiration.
— The method is immediately available when most needed, for example at the scene of a drowning accident, electrocution in the home, etc.

The method is made easier if a Safar or Brook airway is available but on no account must mouth-to-mouth breathing be delayed when these airways are not immediately available. The doctor has his own 'apparatus' in the form of lungs, mouth and hands.

EXTERNAL CARDIAC MASSAGE OR COMPRESSION

The technique is very simple and can easily be learned. Essentially it comprises intermittent compression of the heart between the mobile sternum in front and the thoracic vertebrae behind (Fig. 12.3). By virtue of the valvular arrangement of the heart, blood is expelled into the aorta and the pulmonary arteries following each compression (artificial systole). On releasing the sternum the heart fills with blood again (artificial diastole) from the great veins (inferior and superior venae cavae) and the pulmonary veins. The heart is compressed in a cephalad (headwards) direction and not

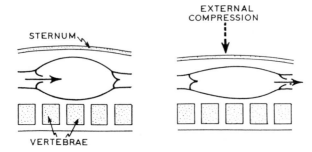

Fig. 12.3 This figure shows how the technique of external cardiac massage works. When pressure is applied to the sternum the blood is driven from the heart into the circulation. On release of sternal pressure the heart refills with venous blood in readiness for the next stroke.

sideways, this latter movement being prevented by the firm attachment of the pericardium.

The following are the simple steps which make up the manœuvre:

— Note the time and clear the airway. Assist ventilation if the patient is not breathing, either by the mouth-to-mouth method or with a resuscitator if one is available.

— Place the patient on his back on a firm surface, for example the floor, or insert fracture boards if in bed. A soft bed prevents effective massage.

— Place one hand palm down over the lower third of the sternum.

— The heel of the other hand is now used on top of the lower hand to compress the chest wall intermittently. The correct motion is almost a blow but with a squeezing action on the 'follow-through'.

— Repeat this sternal compression 60–80 times/minute.

— In children it is sufficient to compress the sternum with the fingers of one hand only, to avoid undue force and damage to the chest wall.

— External cardiac massage is futile unless spontaneous breathing is present and adequate, or assisted ventilation is performed simultaneously.

The blood which this operation circulates *must* be oxygenated in the lungs to be of value. A ratio of 4 sternal compressions to 1 inflation of the lungs is recommended.

On the rare occasion when the doctor or nurse is single handed both assistance to ventilation and external cardiac massage can be performed at the one time.

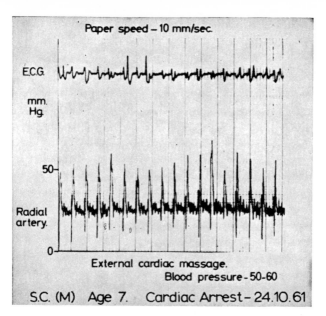

Fig. 12.4 Electrocardiograms during cardiac massage. The upper tracings are of the ECG and the lower tracings of the arterial pressure in the radial artery. The arterial pressure is maintained at 50–60 mmHg by external cardiac massage.

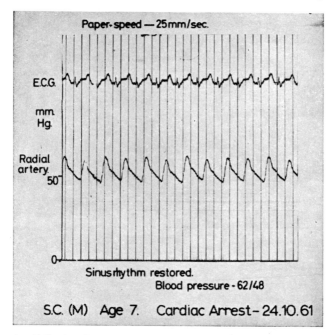

Fig. 12.5 Following the cardiac massage and electrical defibrillation of the heart, normal sinus rhythm can be seen on the ECG. The arterial pressure is 62/48 mmHg.

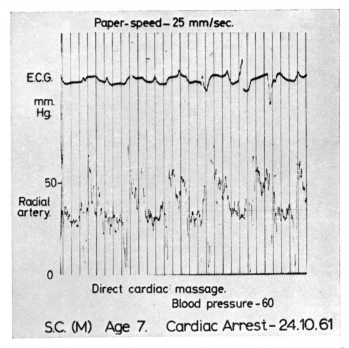

Fig. 12.6 The chest has now been opened and direct cardiac massage started. The arterial pressure is about 60 mmHg.

During this emergency someone other than the person performing the resuscitation must send for the anaesthetist and/or surgeon in charge of the patient. They may decide to continue with the method or may institute direct cardiac massage after a thoracotomy. An ECG will determine whether the heart is arrested in asystole or ventricular fibrillation (Figs. 12.4–12.6). If the latter, then electrical defibrillation will be required either externally or directly on the heart itself.

Signs of successful massage
An immediate improvement in the patient's colour.

Palpable carotid pulses—in time with each sternal compression.

Contraction of the pupils.

The resuscitation must continue until these signs of success are present and adequate spontaneous cardiac action and respiration return or until the doctor in charge indicates that hope is abandoned.

Causes of unsuccessful massage

Inadequate ventilation. This results in poor oxygenation of the blood returning to the heart and going to the brain.

Ineffective massage. Commonly ineffective massage is caused by the subject lying on a soft surface, but occasionally it is unavoidable in thick-chested or obese individuals. Direct massage is more effective in the latter case.

To give an indication of the efficacy of this technique it should be sufficient to mention Kouwenhoven's* original series of 20 patients of all ages. Systolic arterial pressures of 60–100 mmHg were attained during external cardiac massage with more than 50 per cent long-term survival.

Cardiac arrest chart

Although there is no substitute for a thorough and continuing programme of instruction in resuscitation techniques for all medical, nursing and ancillary staff, it is generally agreed that a chart outlining the steps to be taken in an emergency is a useful aid. Such a chart includes alternative instructions for the different situations which may be encountered and guidance as to the necessary drugs and their dosage. The cardiac arrest chart should be available in all casualty departments and operating theatres and a copy should be attached to the mobile resuscitation trolley. An example of a cardiac arrest chart is included on p. 186.

* Kouwenhoven, W. B., Jude, J. R. & Knickerbocker, G. G. (1960) 'Closed-chest cardiac massage.' *J.A.M.A.*, **173**, 1064.

MANAGEMENT OF CARDIAC ARREST

DON'T waste time. You have only 3 minutes to establish circulation.

DON'T give drugs until type and cause of arrest is determined.

DON'T wait for ECG to begin treatment. An absent BP and absent pulse in a major vessel means cardiac arrest.

INITIAL EMERGENCY

1. Note the time.
2. Commence external cardiac massage immediately on firm surface.
3. Commence assistance to ventilation if necessary.
   (Mouth-to-mouth breathing or bellows resuscitator.)
4. Send for resuscitation team and trolley.
   (Trolley carries ECG, defibrillator, etc.)

DUTIES OF RESUSCITATION TEAM

(**Note:** In many cases the entire procedure can be followed without thoracotomy. Only if there is no response to the external methods is the chest opened.)

ANAESTHETIST

1. Establish a clear airway, e.g. endotracheal tube.
2. Ventilate lungs with 100% oxygen.
3. Tilt patient's head down 15 degrees.
4. Check carotid pulse when cardiac massage is established.
5. Check BP.
6. Set up intravenous infusion as vehicle for drugs.

SURGEON

1. Continue external cardiac massage.
2. Apply external defibrillator electrodes if indicated.
3. If direct massage or internal defibrillation is indicated perform thoracotomy, i.e. open left 4th interspace transversely from sternal margin to mid-axillary line.

ASSISTANT

1. Connect ECG leads to patient, confirm diagnosis, and observe ECG constantly.
2. Stand-by to relieve surgeon performing massage.
3. Operate defibrillation equipment if required.

NURSES

1. Assist anaesthetist with emergency syringes and transfusion equipment.
2. Keep note of time and events.
3. Assist surgeon if thoracotomy is performed.

MANAGEMENT OF CARDIAC ARREST

POSSIBLE SITUATIONS EXISTING AFTER ADEQUATE MASSAGE AND OXYGENATION

1. THE HEART RESUMES A NORMAL BEAT

(a) Continue massage in rhythm with beat until the BP is maintained at a minimum of 80 mmHg systolic.

(b) If contractions do not improve give adrenaline 1:1000, 0.5–1 ml (diluted to 10 ml with sterile water) into the cavity of the right ventricle.

(c) If contractions are fairly good but BP remains low, give 2–4 mg isoprenaline in 500 ml 5% glucose slowly intravenously.

(d) In all cases give sodium bicarbonate intravenously to correct acidosis (100 mmol for the average adult).

(e) If thoracotomy has been performed close chest with adequate haemostasis and water-seal drain.

2. THE HEART REMAINS IN ARREST

(A) The heart is in fibrillation

(a) Carry out electrical defibrillation external or internal and continue adequate massage between shocks.

(b) Administer sodium bicarbonate intravenously to correct acidosis (100 mmol for average adult).

(c) If spontaneous beat returns follow column 1.

(d) If heart is in asystole follow column 2B.

(B) The heart is in asystole

(a) Continue adequate massage.

(b) Give calcium chloride 10%, 5–10 ml, intravenously or into the cavity of the right ventricle.

(c) Give sodium bicarbonate intravenously to correct acidosis (100 mmol for average adult).

(d) If asystole persists give adrenaline 1:1000, 0.5–1 ml (diluted to 10 ml with sterile water) into cavity of right ventricle.

(e) If heart beat returns follow column 1.

(f) If asystole persists continue massage up to one hour or until heart fails to fill in diastole.

13

Anaesthesia in obstetrics

The administration of anaesthetics in obstetric cases has many hazards, since two separate patients, the mother and the child, have to be considered. Not infrequently, the fact that an anaesthetic is required at all for some operative procedure is also an indication that neither the mother nor the child is in the best of condition for anaesthesia. Many of the indications for Caesarean section and even for forceps delivery are those involving some condition adversely affecting the fetus; for instance antepartum haemorrhage, where the placental circulation is interfered with, or prolonged labour, where there has been undue compression of the fetus, are likely causes of hypoxia in the child. In addition, the mother may be suffering from some complication of pregnancy and may have a full or semi-full stomach. The large pregnant uterus embarrasses respiration and the position on the table required for some procedures, for example forceps deliveries, is such that respiration is further embarrassed.

Before passing to the consideration of the anaesthetic techniques used in obstetric practice, it is desirable to give some attention to the problems of providing pain relief during normal labour.

Provision of analgesia during labour
Labour is divided into three stages, the first stage up to full dilatation of the cervix, the second stage from then until the child is delivered, and the third till the placenta is delivered.

During the early stage of labour when the contractions of the uterus are felt as discomfort rather than pain, it is traditional to use mild sedatives to control this discomfort. In some patients where anxiety is present the use of small doses of a tranquilliser or barbiturate may be tried. It is, however, essential to remember that when using a barbiturate in the presence of pain in such cases, excitement and restlessness may be produced.

The regular severe contractions, felt as definite and increasing pains, are usually controlled by the administration of a more potent analgesic drug. The one most favoured is pethidine, given in doses of 100 mg intramuscularly. Morphine, which is an effective analgesic and provides some degree of sedation also, has fallen from favour because of the respiratory depression which it may cause and the likelihood that this might interfere with the onset of spontaneous breathing by the baby. It is now believed that the degree of respiratory depression produced by pethidine is almost as great as that produced by morphine, in the equivalent dosage. Pethidine is, however, claimed to facilitate dilatation of the cervix during labour and its lack of sedative properties and production of respiratory depression have been overcome in two ways.

To enhance its sedative properties it may be given with a phenothiazine drug, such as promazine, and this combination has been used with apparently favourable results by some obstetricians. To overcome the respiratory depression which it causes, pethidine has been mixed with the antagonist drug levallorphan. The value of this combination is questioned by some and, if an antagonist drug is required, it may be better to administer it separately either to the patient or to the child after delivery. Nalorphine (Lethidrone) or naloxone (Narcan) may be used for this purpose.

The objections to the use of the non-volatile sedative or analgesic agents, because they produce depression of the fetus, can be minimised by restricting their use to the early part of labour, that is before the cervix is fully dilated. From then on until the child is delivered it is customary to use volatile or gaseous analgesic agents, which are rapidly excreted by the mother and should cause minimal fetal depression. The two possibilities are that nitrous oxide in oxygen is inhaled or that low concentrations of trichloroethylene in air are used. In this country, midwives may administer nitrous oxide with 50 per cent oxygen, and trichloroethylene or methoxyflurane from specially designed inhalers.

It is possible to combine nitrous oxide and oxygen premixed in one cylinder (Entonox) such that it will normally be delivered in the same proportions and supplied on demand. If the cylinder has been exposed to severe cold—and many cylinders are stored outside even in winter—the gases may separate and when the cylinder is almost empty lower proportions of oxygen are supplied. This can be prevented by inverting the cylinders several times before use. A special demand valve is used with the cylinder and the complete Entonox unit is shown in use in Figure 13.1.

Trichloroethylene may be administered in 0.35 or 0.5 per cent concentrations in air from temperature-compensated vaporisers

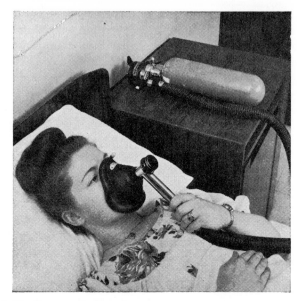

Fig. 13.1 The Entonox apparatus in use.

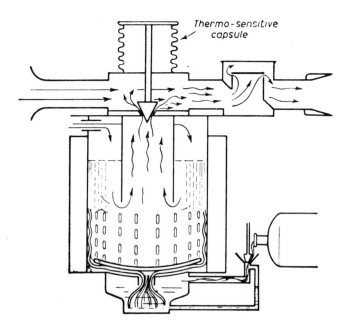

Fig. 13.2 Diagram illustrating the principle of the Emotril inhaler.

which ensure that the percentage is constant under all circumstances, and this is a considerable step forward in this technique. Figure 13.2 illustrates the working principles of the Emotril inhaler. An inhaler working on similar lines to produce up to 0.5 per cent methoxyflurane (Fig. 13.3) has been used with equally good results.

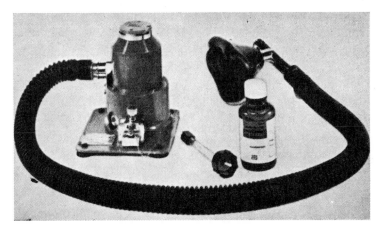

Fig. 13.3 The Cardiff inhaler.

The use of these volatile or gaseous analgesics, from the stage of dilatation of the cervix to delivery of the child, is facilitated by the previous administration of the nonvolatile agents which have been described. This is particularly valuable where nitrous oxide and oxygen is to be administered as the residual effects of opiate or pethidine administration supplements the weak analgesic properties of these agents. The patient should have had antenatal instruction in the use of the analgesic apparatus and be told to take deep breaths of the mixture with the onset of the first pain.

Increasing use is being made of extradural blockade to obtain pain relief during labour. This is not only valuable in relieving pain but in allowing the cervix to dilate. Combined with oxytocin infusions to accelerate labour continuous epidural blockade is becoming increasingly popular where adequate trained staff are available.

Hypnosis and relaxation exercises
The teachings of Dr Grantly Dick Read regarding the value of relaxation during childbirth have been fairly widely accepted. Antenatal classes, where the patient is taught the technique of

relaxation to be practised during the actual childbirth, are now common practice. This voluntary control and relaxation of specific muscle groups is undoubtedly of value and in many patients gives considerable relief from the pains of labour. Similarly many practitioners have found the use of hypnosis, when induced in the antenatal period and practised by the patient during labour, to be of considerable value. Hypnosis has undoubtedly some applications in this field—and some potential dangers—but when used by skilled hypnotists it undoubtedly produces good results in selected patients. It is not, however, generally considered to be an adequate substitute for other forms of analgesia.

ANAESTHETIC AND ANALGESIC TECHNIQUES IN OPERATIVE OBSTETRICS

We may summarise the problems presented by the obstetric patient as follows:
1. The stomach is frequently full.
2. The position adopted for delivery is such that respiration is hampered.
3. In any event respiration is restricted by the presence of the pregnant uterus.
4. The depressant effect of analgesics on the fetus must be borne in mind.
5. The obstetrician, in his manipulations, may cause further embarrassment to respiration and may cause the patient to vomit or regurgitate.
6. Many patients and their babies are in poor condition when anaesthesia has to be induced.

There are many ways of overcoming these problems during operative obstetrics. The first is to employ, where possible, some form of *local analgesia.*

Infiltration analgesia is suitable for the performance of an episiotomy or suturing the perineum after delivery. Attention must be paid to the dose employed, as the perineum at this stage is very vascular and absorption of the local analgesic from the area may be very rapid. Only dilute solutions of the chosen analgesic are required.

Pudendal block, described in Chapter 16, is suitable for a low forceps delivery and may be carried out in private homes. It is a technique which should be mastered by anyone carrying out single-handed obstetrics, as it is probably the safest technique for use in these circumstances, although it may be rather more uncomfortable for the patient than the use of a general anaesthetic. It is perhaps significant that pudendal block is the anaesthetic of choice in many obstetric hospitals and its more widespread use outside hospital is to be recommended.

Extradural (epidural) analgesia

This method may have been used during the earlier stages of labour and with a catheter in the epidural space it is possible to extend its use for operative procedures. If epidural blockade has not been used before it may be instituted at this stage using the techniques described on page 220. It has largely replaced paracervical block for forceps delivery because of the adverse effects the latter technique may have on the fetus. Extradural analgesia is especially valuable in cases of cervical dystocia.

Subarachnoid block (spinal analgesia)

This form of analgesia has been widely used for years, particularly for low forceps deliveries and for Caesarean section. It is not now a popular method of analgesia for the latter procedure. The use of subarachnoid analgesia may be associated with a fall in blood pressure which may be harmful and, if the injection spreads too far headwards, then the action of the intercostal muscles may be impaired. This is particularly dangerous where the diaphragm is splinted by the large uterus and respiratory embarrassment has been noted. This has been cited as a cause of death during the performance of caesarean section under spinal analgesia. In addition, it has been pointed out that the uterus contracts after a spinal has been given and that this may interfere with placental circulation if an unduly long time elapses between the induction of analgesia and delivery of the baby.

General anaesthesia

In most hospitals general anaesthesia is used for operative obstetrics. The hazards associated with induction of anaesthesia in the presence of a full stomach are those which have been noted previously. Routine antacid therapy in the form of tablets given 2-hourly during labour will do much to keep the stomach contents alkaline, thus avoiding the hazards of the acid aspiration syndrome (p. 116). This is more pleasant than the single dose of 15 ml of, for example, magnesium trisilicate which, though unpalatable in a parched patient, will otherwise be indicated. Where possible the stomach should be emptied before induction of anaesthesia. This may be contra-indicated in cases of antepartum haemorrhage, where the retching associated with passing an oesophageal tube may cause further bleeding.

The patient should be placed in the left lateral position as for a forceps delivery in the classical Sims' position and anaesthesia induced and an endotracheal tube passed. Even if a tube is not to be passed, anaesthesia may still be induced in this position.

In any event the bed or the theatre table must be capable of tilting in any direction, so that either a head-up or head-down position can be adopted if necessary. It need hardly be stressed that, as in outpatient anaesthesia, all the normal apparatus to be found in the general operating theatre should be present in the obstetric department, namely an efficient suction apparatus, bronchoscope, anaesthetic machine and a full range of drugs and endotracheal tubes.

The choice of agents used for obstetric anaesthesia varies from centre to centre but, at present, a combination very widely used is thiopentone, suxamethonium, nitrous oxide and oxygen. Pre-medication is usually with atropine or hyoscine only, to avoid fetal depression. In some centres diazepam has been employed to avoid awareness during anaesthesia. After pre-oxygenation anaesthesia is induced with a small dose of thiopentone, up to 250 mg and suxamethonium, 50 mg, is injected through the same needle. A cuffed tracheal tube is passed and inflation of the lungs carried out with nitrous oxide and at least 33 per cent of oxygen. The use of high minute volumes up to 14 litres/minute for 3–4 minutes will again reduce the incidence of awareness during anaesthesia as it takes time to clear nitrogen from the lungs. Intermittent injections of suxamethonium or a longer-acting relaxant such as curare are given to facilitate controlled ventilation and normally no more potent analgesic is used until after delivery of the child. From then on intravenous or volatile agents may be administered. This technique is applicable to forceps deliveries, Caesarean sections and other obstetric manœuvres, the hazards of a full stomach being present in each. Where uterine relaxation is desirable the administration of halothane for a short time may be useful.

The use of more potent volatile anaesthetic agents such as diethyl-ether and halothane and the gaseous anaesthetic cyclopropane is not popular nowadays because of the effect on the fetus and on the uterus. Halothane, in particular, causes uterine relaxation and may cause considerable postpartum haemorrhage if administered in any quantity. It may however be given in concentrations of not more than 0.5 per cent and is widely used to supplement nitrous oxide and oxygen in an attempt to avoid awareness. It is claimed that at this concentration blood loss is not increased during delivery.

Despite this a nitrous oxide–oxygen–ether sequence was used for years in most obstetric units. In an emergency a practitioner familiar with this type of anaesthetic is probably safer to employ it for his obstetric patients. Most anaesthetists, however, consider that the thiopentone, relaxant, nitrous oxide–oxygen sequence, where possible, is the better technique.

This important sub-specialty of anaesthesia can be seen to present many special problems to the anaesthetist and is worthy of detailed and separate consideration. The student is referred for further information on the subject to Moir, D. (1976) *Obstetric Anaesthesia and Analgesia*. London: Baillière Tindall.

14

Anaesthesia for the outpatient

Anaesthetics for outpatients present considerable problems. Many of the patients who are subjected to these anaesthetics are unprepared and may have attended at the hospital only a short time before if at all. Often they may have a full stomach and only rarely have they had premedication. In addition, if recovery facilities are limited, the anaesthetist has to attempt to administer an anaesthetic from which there will be a rapid and complete recovery. This latter requirement is sometimes incompatible with providing ideal operating conditions for the surgeon in large, husky, patients.

Given adequate facilities for preparing the patients and a modicum of recovery beds in which the patients may lie until the full recovery of consciousness and reflex activity, the anaesthetist can do a great deal. However, even in the absence of these conditions he should endeavour to provide the same safety as he would for an inpatient in the hospital, a matter which may demand considerable ingenuity.

In cases with a *full stomach* the operation should be postponed until four hours after the patient last had anything to eat or drink. Where the operation is not an absolute emergency and the patient can be trusted, he may be asked to return to the hospital later on in the day if he has not come from a distance. Alternatively, active measures should be taken to empty the stomach by means of a stomach tube or oesophageal tube or as may be indicated. Administration of 15 ml of an antacid may again be of value. It is important to remember that in many of these patients the state of the stomach may depend on the interval between the last meal and the time of accident. Thus, although a meal may have been eaten or fluid taken many hours before, if the injury has been sustained within an hour or so of the meal, the stomach may still be full a long time afterwards. This is true even in cases with injuries to the limbs with no abdominal injuries, and if forgotten is a cause of trouble and sometimes even death during anaesthesia for a relatively trivial procedure. The hazards of anaesthesia in the presence of a full stomach are unrelated to the severity of the operation to be performed.

It need hardly be said that, when an anaesthetic is undertaken in the outpatient department, the normal precautions associated with the administration of an anaesthetic anywhere else should be employed. This means that suction apparatus, complete with suction catheters, a laryngoscope, endotracheal tubes and an emergency bronchoscope should be readily available. A full range of drugs, thiopentone, relaxants, inhalational agents and the drugs normally available for cardiac arrest should be easily available.

Premedication is normally omitted. The use of sedative premedication in the patient who is to go home is unwise, as this delays the recovery of consciousness and will make the patient unsteady on his feet after the effects of the anaesthetic itself have worn off. It is often not possible to administer atropine one hour before the anaesthetic and it may have to be given intravenously, immediately before induction. The need for atropine is considerably reduced where non-irritant anaesthetics are used.

The anaesthetic technique which is employed, in patients who have a full stomach and in whom passage of a tube cannot guarantee complete emptying, will depend on the skill and judgment of the anaesthetist concerned. The specialist anaesthetist may pre-oxygenate his patient, tilt him head upwards to prevent regurgitation of stomach content and induce anaesthesia with thiopentone or propanidid and suxamethonium, apply cricoid pressure and pass a cuffed endotracheal tube. This technique is relatively safe in the hands of the skilled anaesthetist who can guarantee to introduce a cuffed endotracheal tube under most circumstances. However, for the beginner, this technique is a risky one and he is advised to select other means.

Anaesthesia may be induced by inhalation agents such as nitrous oxide, oxygen and diethylether. If this is done the patient retains his cough reflex during the early stages of induction and should he vomit he is less liable to inhale foreign matter. An additional safety factor may be to induce anaesthesia with the patient in the lateral position so that if vomiting does take place, the vomitus will trickle out of the mouth. This is not so difficult as it might seem and is a technique which is worthy of more attention.

It is worth stressing that even when a local analgesic has to be given, the danger of the full stomach cannot be ignored for, unless minute doses of local analgesic are being given, one must always bear in mind the possibility of an adverse reaction to the drug taking place, namely the occurrence of convulsions or circulatory collapse. In the former case the treatment of this condition is to administer intravenous thiopentone or a relaxant. Here the danger of vomiting and regurgitation is as great as during a general anaesthetic. However, where the stomach is full and a local analgesic can be used in small quantities this is probably a good technique to employ (Chapter 16).

During inhalational anaesthesia in outpatients, it is possible to use a transparent mask so that vomited and regurgitated material can be seen at the earliest opportunity, and one should never under any circumstances strap the mask on to the patient's face when the state of the stomach is not known with certainty.

Rapid recovery of consciousness is essential in outpatient anaesthetic procedures. Often the patient is required to leave the outpatient department soon after the anaesthetic and he should do so in as co-ordinated a state as possible. Generally this means that thiopentone is not used or, if it is, only in the smallest doses. An alternative is to use methohexitone, propanidid or Althesin from which the recovery is more rapid and complete than after thiopentone. Many anaesthetists, however, do not use intravenous agents at all in outpatients and prefer nitrous oxide, oxygen and halothane or induce anaesthesia with a 50 per cent mixture of cyclopropane in oxygen as described on pages 86 and 201.

The use of short-acting muscle relaxants, such as suxamethonium, is popular with many anaesthetists in that fractures may be manipulated under very light anaesthesia from which recovery of consciousness is fairly rapid. Simple fractures of the forearm and leg may be dealt with in this way. However, the danger of using suxamethonium in a patient with a full stomach must never be forgotten nor must the incidence of severe post-operative muscular pains. These are similar to those of influenza, with an incidence of up to perhaps 50 per cent, which discounts many of the advantages of light anaesthesia. Their incidence may be reduced where propanidid is used to induce anaesthesia, although the period of apnoea following suxamethonium may be prolonged after the administration of propanidid.

After the outpatient has recovered from his anaesthetic, particularly when he has had a barbiturate, care should be taken to ensure that he is sent home under supervision. In particular, he must not be allowed to drive his car home although at the time he may feel quite capable of driving. When sitting in the erect position for a period behind the wheel, he may find that he is not capable of handling a car in traffic, the medico-legal consequences of which are obvious.

In conclusion, it must be emphasised that the anaesthetic for minor operations in the outpatient must never be treated lightly, since serious complications and even death are almost as likely to follow as they are in the inpatient. As many outpatients treated for minor complaints are fit and healthy, serious anaesthetic accidents are all the more tragic.

It has been said that minor surgery can be made perfect by treating each operation with the care that one would devote to a major operation. The same can be said for the simplest anaesthetic; it can be made safe only by employing the full precautions one would for administering an anaesthetic for a major procedure.

15

Anaesthesia for dental surgery

In the United Kingdom, more general anaesthetics are given for dental procedures than are given in all the hospitals in the country for other types of surgery.

Anaesthesia for dental surgery is a procedure which many occasional anaesthetists are called upon to undertake. In this book, the subject will be dealt with only in outline, because a simple description of the techniques is no substitute for practical experience. Competent dental anaesthesia, perhaps more than any other type of anaesthetic practice, is an art.

Assessment
Many of the problems associated with anaesthetising dental patients are those which are found in the outpatients described in the previous chapter. However, many of the patients come by appointment and can be presumed to arrive with an empty stomach. Some, a few of whom may have been extremely nervous, will have received mild sedation from their dentist and this should be ascertained before commencing anaesthesia. The anaesthetist should always question the patient regarding his general medical history, particularly about untoward consequences of previous dental anaesthesia. It is essential also to be aware of any recent or current drug therapy. Full routine physical examination is desirable and it is regrettable that, in many types of dental anaesthetic practice, this may be impracticable.

Position
Most dental patients are anaesthetised in the dental chair and the hazards of the sitting-up position have been dealt with in considerable detail by Bourne. He claims that in this position the patient may suffer a vasovagal attack with hypotension and faint. The results of this can be minimised by lowering the back of the chair so that the patient is in a semi-recumbent position. Ideally, however, the operation should be carried out in the supine position.

Anaesthesia

Nitrous oxide is administered with adequate amounts of oxygen and a volatile supplement, normally halothane. A nasal mask such as that shown in Figure 15.1 may be used to induce anaesthesia. A mouth 'gag' or prop is inserted between the teeth, and a pack is inserted into the mouth posteriorly but not so far back as to obstruct the nasopharynx through which breathing takes place. The pack is essential not only to prevent dilution of the anaesthetic mixture by air but to prevent inhalation of blood and debris from the mouth during the anaesthetic. Older dental anaesthetic machines, incorporating an intermittent flow principle, with mixing valves for oxygen and nitrous oxide, should be regarded with caution since the oxygen concentration may be less than the nominal value.

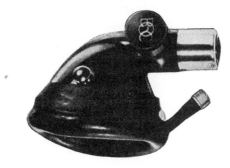

Fig. 15.1 Nasal mask

Present practice favours the standard continuous flow anaesthetic machines. Bourne has drawn attention to a number of cases where recovery of consciousness has been very slow and mental impairment has followed, suggesting that cerebral hypoxia has occurred with consequent brain damage. This may be attributable to inadvertent obstruction of the airway, in spite of an appropriate inspired oxygen concentration. A mixture of nitrous oxide and oxygen alone for dental anaesthesia is seldom used except perhaps during extraction of a single anterior tooth in a child.

Induction of anaesthesia with cyclopropane and oxygen has been advocated by Bourne. Initially, he suggested the use of 50 per cent cyclopropane and 50 per cent oxygen, but it was shown that this might be inflammable if a spark resulted from forceps being applied to teeth, and the mixture has been diluted now by the introduction of nitrogen. The reservoir bag is filled with this mixture and the patient is allowed to breathe through a mask.

When anaesthesia has been established, and this takes place after about a dozen breaths, a gag and throat pack are inserted as before and anaesthesia is maintained with halothane in a mixture of 66 per cent nitrous oxide in oxygen.

Halothane as a supplement to nitrous oxide and oxygen anaesthesia has become popular for the induction of anaesthesia in several centres; when anaesthesia is established, it may be maintained if necessary through a nasal mask using the nitrous oxide–oxygen–halothane mixture. However, it is standard practice in adults to induce anaesthesia with a small dose of an intravenous agent: methohexitone, Althesin or propanidid. Anaesthesia is then maintained with the inhalation agents described previously. As with all outpatient procedures, adequate facilities for recovery and the return of the patient to his home must be available.

Cardiac arrhythmia during dental extractions has been demonstrated and it is considered that ventricular fibrillation or asystole may be a cause of the unexpected deaths which occur during dental anaesthesia. The value of atropine and other agents in preventing this is a matter of debate but it is generally accepted that infiltration round the base of a difficult tooth with a local analgesic is a valuable prophylactic procedure.

ANALGESIA FOR CONSERVATIVE DENTAL TREATMENT

In some patients, conservative dental procedures can be carried out more easily when the patient is sedated. To this end, some anaesthetists and dentists favour techniques whereby intermittent intravenous injections of sedatives such as diazepam are given to produce a calm patient while the dental procedures are carried out under local analgesia. During these procedures, the patient breathes air and a clear airway must be maintained while treatment is carried out.

It is considered that since any general anaesthetic carries a risk, local analgesia by infiltration or nerve block should be used where possible.

Major dental procedures should be undertaken under endotracheal anaesthesia in the same way as for any other operation on the head and neck.

If a patient is a poor anaesthetic risk for medical reasons, he should be admitted to hospital.

Finally, we would emphasise that practical training in dental anaesthesia is a post-graduate study to be undertaken at the hands of experts. It is our hope that such knowledge may be gained from the appropriate chapters in this book and that dental anaesthesia, while having special problems of its own, would be based on the principles that underlie good anaesthetic practice in other fields. Further detailed descriptions of the problems involved and the methods of overcoming them will be found in Green, R. A. & Coplans, M. P. (1973) *Anaesthesia and Analgesia in Dentistry*, London: Lewis.

16

Selected local and regional techniques

The advent of the muscle relaxants caused a comparative neglect of certain well-tried and useful methods of local and regional analgesia. These techniques demand a precise knowledge of anatomy and this may also explain some of their unpopularity. Recently some of these local and regional methods have enjoyed a deserved return to popularity. Before detailing the actual methods employed it would be well to consider briefly their advantages and potential hazards.

A common misconception is that a local or regional technique is a completely safe alternative to general anaesthesia in patients who have eaten immediately before being admitted for emergency surgery. This dangerous notion must be disposed of at the outset, since there is no guarantee that the anaesthetist will not be confronted with a toxic reaction following injection of the analgesic solution.

All patients presented for anaesthesia, local, regional or general, should be fully prepared in the normal manner wherever possible. Nervous patients will usually benefit from preliminary light sedation with a suitable agent. Generally speaking it is unwise to attempt these procedures in restless or drunken patients since a violent movement, when the needle is introduced to perform say a brachial plexus block, can have disastrous results, for example intravascular injection.

Despite the potential hazards these techniques have definite advantages to offer. They are:

— The minimum of equipment is required.
— The patient can if desired remain conscious and co-operative.
— General anaesthesia can be avoided in patients with gross respiratory or cardiovascular disease.
— In many instances a 'dry field' can be provided for the surgeon either by vasoconstriction, when adrenaline has been added to the analgesic solution or, in the regional techniques, by posturing the patient following the sympathetic blockade.

—Prolonged post-operative epidural analgesia can be provided by continuing the analgesia with incremental doses via an indwelling catheter.

LOCAL ANALGESIC AGENTS

The drugs used as local analgesic agents vary widely in their chemical composition, some being hydroxy compounds, such as the long-acting benzyl alcohol; others, including procaine, are esters of aromatic acids while the remainder are a miscellaneous group including the widely used lignocaine.

The mode of action of the commonly used local analgesics is discussed in Chapter 1. Being stored as water-soluble salts, usually the hydrochloride, with a low pH, they react with the alkaline tissues (pH 7.4) to liberate free base thus—

$$LA : HCl + OH \rightarrow LA + Cl + H_2O$$
$$\text{(free base)}$$

The effect of this free base on the nerve is to stop conduction of impulses along it. This is the main effect and ideally the only one which should follow injection of these agents.

Side effects and toxic effects

Side effects are often noticeable after injection of local analgesic agents into the tissues or the epidural or subarachnoid spaces. It has been shown that the agent used can be detected in the blood, even in the absence of intravascular injection, and this results in a central action and the production of the unwanted effects. These are usually limited to a feeling of warmth and perhaps drowsiness due to peripheral vasodilatation and central depression. If the patient sits or stands up he may feel faint.

Toxic effects may be manifest as restlessness, anxiety and confusion followed by twitchings, often proceeding to convulsions—the stage of cerebral stimulation. This may cause death by asphyxia, or may be followed by central nervous system depression with unconsciousness, respiratory depression and fall in blood pressure. These effects are due to the central action of the drug on the brain.

Sometimes, however, cardiovascular collapse may follow massive intravascular injection of the local analgesic. This is a result of direct action on the heart or blood vessels.

Treatment. At the stage of anxiety or slight twitching a small dose of a short-acting barbiturate may be given carefully and slowly. Oxygen should also be given.

If the patient has convulsed a short-acting muscle relaxant (suxamethonium 50 mg) should be administered intravenously and controlled ventilation with oxygen commenced. The trachea should be intubated to prevent soiling of the lungs with gastric contents. A barbiturate is contra-indicated when convulsions have developed, as circulatory depression, if not already present, would follow and be aggravated by the barbiturate.

Cardiovascular collapse is treated with vasopressors, plasma infusion and if necessary cardiac massage.

Prevention of toxic effects

Toxic effects are caused by *overdosage, intravascular injection* or *idiosyncrasy of the patient* to the normal dose of the drug.

Idiosyncrasy is rare and *intravascular injection* can be avoided by frequent aspiration through the needle and by keeping the needle point moving during injection.

Overdosage, the most important of the three, is worthy of further consideration. There is a maximum safe dose for each local analgesic drug beyond which toxic effects will be produced. In this respect local analgesics are no different from other drugs, but failure to remember this simple fact is a frequent cause of trouble. The safe dose of a local analgesic varies with:

The drug used—lignocaine is twice as potent as procaine.

The strength of solution—the stronger solution is more rapidly absorbed and causes toxic effects more rapidly. For healthy adults (70 kg) we may use procaine thus:

$$200 \text{ ml of } 0.5 \text{ per cent} = 1000 \text{ mg}$$
$$75 \text{ ml of } 1.0 \text{ per cent} = 750 \text{ mg}$$
$$25 \text{ ml of } 2.0 \text{ per cent} = 500 \text{ mg}$$

The patient. As with other drugs reduced dosage is required in frail patients.

Site of injection. Absorption is rapid from vascular areas, for example the perineum, and it is claimed that from inflamed mucosae absorption is almost as rapid as that following intravenous injection.

Hyaluronidase. This increases absorption by promoting the spread of the drug in the tissues.

Adrenaline by delaying absorption, allows a larger dose of local analgesic to be given.

A consideration of these six factors and the extent to which they apply in any individual will be valuable in establishing the maximum dose of the local analgesic agent which can be given to each patient.

The drugs used
There are a large number of local analgesic agents available and basically they all produce their main effect—local analgesia—and side effects as described in the preceding pages. Six agents are considered in greater detail.

Cocaine, the first local analgesic used in clinical anaesthetic practice, is a vasoconstrictor unlike the other agents. It is effective by injection and surface application but is extremely toxic—four times more so than procaine. Its use is now limited to topical application for ophthalmic and ear, nose and throat procedures in a diminishing number of hospitals.

Procaine (*Novocaine, Planocaine*) was the most widely used drug in local analgesia until recently. Rapidly metabolised and only one-quarter as toxic as cocaine, it is used by injection but is not absorbed through mucous membranes except in excessive concentrations. It is therefore valueless for topical analgesia.

It has been used intravenously as an analgesic for burns dressings, to control itching and as a supplement to nitrous oxide and oxygen in patients who have received a myoneural blocking drug and who are being ventilated artificially. In addition it has been used intravenously and intrapericardially to control cardiac arrhythmias during cardiac surgery.

Great care must be employed when giving procaine intravenously as toxic effects are easily produced. This is a method for the expert.

Lignocaine (*Xylocaine, Lidocaine, Duncaine, Xylotox*). In most centres this drug has replaced procaine. It is very stable, being little affected by heat, acids, alkalis or prolonged storage. It diffuses well, has a rapid onset of action and a more prolonged action than procaine. It is also an excellent surface analgesic. While it was originally claimed that the maximum dose was the same as that of procaine it is now recommended that no more than 200 mg without, and 500 mg with adrenaline should be used in a fit 70 kg

adult (= 1000 mg procaine). Lignocaine 0.5 per cent is equi-analgesic with 2 per cent procaine and 0.25 per cent is adequate for
infiltration. Used in this way lignocaine is a safe and valuable
agent.

Table 16.1 Duration of action and dosage

Drug	Dose		Duration of action	
	Without adrenaline	With adrenaline	Without adrenaline	With adrenaline
Procaine	500 mg	1000 mg	30 min	1–1½ h
Lignocaine	200 mg	500 mg	1 h	2 h
Prilocaine	400 mg	600 mg	1 h	2 h
Bupivacaine	100 mg	150 mg	5 h	No significant prolongation of action
Etidocaine	100 mg	200 mg	5h	No significant prolongation of action

Prilocaine (Citanest) is claimed to be 40 per cent less toxic than
lignocaine, to cause less vasodilatation and to be more rapidly
metabolised. However, in addition to the other side effects of local
analgesics, with doses in excess of 600 mg (the maximum recommended dose), methaemoglobinaemia may occur. This can be
treated if necessary by intravenous injection of methylene blue in
equal dosage, but is a limiting factor to the more widespread use
of this drug.

Bupivacaine (Marcain) is distinguished from the other local analgesic agents in common use mainly by its much greater duration
of action. It would appear to be no more toxic than these other
agents. In a 0.5 per cent concentration containing 1 : 200 000
adrenaline this drug has proved extremely effective for 'single-
shot' extradural blockade in general surgical and obstetrical procedures, giving good analgesia for up to five hours.

Etidocaine (Duranest). This is a long-acting drug related to lignocaine. It is stable and can be repeatedly autoclaved. The onset of
action is rapid and the duration of action is similar to bupivacaine although it may be less toxic. Etidocaine may be used in
concentrations of from 0.25 per cent for local infiltration to 1.5
per cent for extradural blockade. Concentrations as low as 0.5 per
cent produce motor blockade. Similarly to bupivacaine, there is
little prolongation of action by the addition of adrenaline although
toxicity is probably reduced.

Use of hyaluronidase

Hyaluronidase (Hyalase) is used as a spreading agent. It is an enzyme which hydrolyses hyaluronic acid and thus speeds diffusion through the interstitial spaces. Its use speeds onset of analgesia and allows a greater area of analgesia to be produced on infiltration with a smaller volume of analgesic solution. It is of value also in plastic surgical procedures where the injected analgesic solution may distort the anatomy of the operative field.

It is not a substitute for the essential anatomical knowledge necessary for nerve blocking. Further, by increasing the rate of absorption of the analgesic it decreases its duration of action and increases the incidence of toxic reactions. It is usual to add 1000–1500 international units of hyaluronidase to the analgesic solution.

Use of adrenaline

Adrenaline in dilute solution (1 : 100 000–1 : 200 000) is an effective vasoconstrictor when injected into the tissues. This is a valuable property when the drug is used with local analgesics as, with the exception of cocaine, they are all vasodilators. Vasoconstriction, by reducing the absorption of the local analgesic agent, prolongs its action and reduces the incidence of toxic effects with a given dose. As the local analgesic drugs inhibit amine oxidase, adrenaline breakdown is also retarded.

Adrenaline is, however, a dangerous substance and must be used with great care.

Locally the vasoconstriction produced may cause ischaemic damage (see p. 241) and systemically it may cause anxiety, restlessness, tachycardia and even ventricular fibrillation and cardiac arrest. These effects can be avoided by using the drug in 1 : 200 000 concentration which is adequate and by limiting the total dose for any one procedure to the equivalent of 0.5 ml of 1 : 1000 solution. Stronger solutions, for example 1 : 80 000, are unnecesary and should be avoided. Adrenaline should never be injected near to an 'end artery', for example at the base of the finger or in the ear, the nose or the penis.

PREPARATION FOR LOCAL OR REGIONAL ANALGESIA

No matter whether the method contemplated is local infiltration or subarachnoid analgesia, certain basic precautions should be considered.

Premedication

Before minor surgical procedures under local or regional analgesia, premedication is not usually necessary. However, in nervous patients or for major procedures some premedication is desirable. A barbiturate is often employed to allay anxiety. These drugs in the dosage employed are ineffective in preventing the twitching and convulsions seen as toxic effects of the local analgesic drugs.

The empty stomach

It is desirable that even before administering a regional analgesic where consciousness is to be retained the stomach should be empty. Where subarachnoid or epidural techniques are to be employed, coughing and clearing the pharynx may be impaired. With less extensive procedures the risk of vomiting or regurgitation must be borne in mind.

The open vein

A wise precaution before embarking on an extensive local or regional block is to secure access to a convenient vein, by the insertion of an indwelling cannula or the setting up of an intravenous infusion. Should a toxic reaction be encountered later during the procedure it is then possible to give an appropriate intravenous medication quickly.

Checking the injection

The person giving the injection should check that he has the correct drug, in the correct strength of solution, and that the volume he intends to inject does not contain an overdose. He should also verify the presence or absence of adrenaline, noting the quantity and strength in the volume to be injected.

Asepsis

Before embarking on an injection the administrator should scrub and, except for minor infiltrations, should don cap, mask, gown and gloves. The site of injection should be prepared and towelled as for an operation.

Explanation

It is helpful and humane to explain to the patient what you are going to do and not subject him to a series of unexpected jabs with a needle. This may cause pain, loss of confidence and a broken needle.

SELECTED LOCAL ANALGESIC TECHNIQUES

The following are some local analgesic techniques in common use. The techniques of brachial plexus block and intravenous local analgesia are suitable for use in the casualty department while pudendal block is of great assistance to the obstetrician. Epidural analgesia has largely replaced subarachnoid or spinal block but, unlike the other techniques described, these latter are confined to specialist anaesthetic practice.

BRACHIAL PLEXUS BLOCK

The plexus is constituted by the anterior primary divisions of C5, C6, C7, C8, T1 with communicating branches from C4 and T2. These nerves first join into three trunks lying in the neck above the clavicle. Behind the clavicle each trunk divides into an anterior

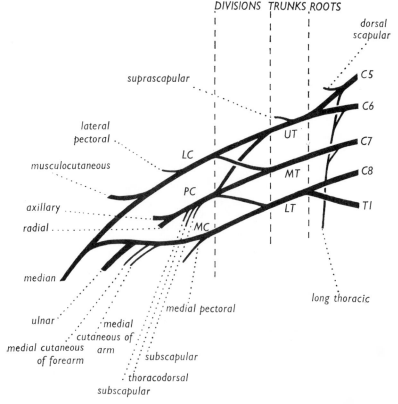

Fig. 16.1 Diagrammatic lay-out of the brachial plexus, UT, MT, LT: upper, middle and lower trunks; LC, PC, MC: lateral, posterior and medial cords.

and posterior division and these unite in the axilla to form three cords (Fig. 16.1). Inferiorly the plexus is related to the first rib, lying between the subclavian artery anteriorly and the scalenus medius behind. Anteriorly the scalenus anterior lies in front of the upper part of the plexus and the clavicle in front of the lower part.

Technique. One of two techniques is commonly used—the supra-clavicular approach or the axillary route. A third approach to the plexus, by the interscalene route, is also used by some clinicians.

The supraclavicular approach

— The patient should be sitting or lying supine with the head rotated to the opposite side and the shoulder, on the side to be blocked, depressed. This can best be accomplished if an assistant applies gentle traction to the hand and arm.
— Following skin preparation with a suitable antiseptic, an in-tradermal wheal is raised 1 cm above the mid-point of the cla-vicle.
— A needle is inserted through the wheal downwards, medially and backwards until paraesthesiae are felt by the patient.

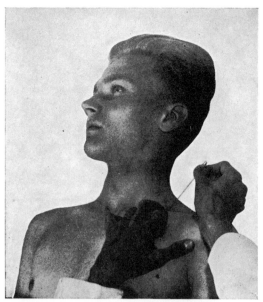

Fig. 16.2 The patient is in the correct position and is shown as he is seen by the anaesthetist. The patient is lying down with a pillow under his shoulders and head. The shoulder of the affected side is depressed, the head is turned to the opposite side and the muscles are relaxed.

— If paraesthesiae are felt, 20–30 ml of 1 per cent lignocaine are
injected following a negative aspiration test.

— If paraesthesiae are not felt, then the needle is inserted until
it contacts the upper surface of the 1st rib and 10 ml of 1 per
cent lignocaine injected following a negative aspiration test.
Three further injections of 10 ml of analgesic solution are made
between the skin and the surface of the 1st rib, each injection
being 1 cm lateral to the preceding one (Figs. 16.2 and 16.3).

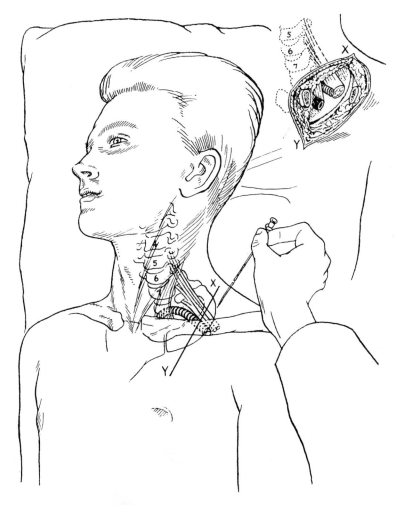

Fig. 16.3 The needle is directed backwards, medially, and downwards towards the
plexus lying on the first rib. *Inset:* An incision along the line XY has been made
and exposes the structures crossing the first rib. The second quarter of the clavicle
has been removed.

If the patient has experienced paraesthesiae before injection the onset of the block is rapid, otherwise 15 minutes may elapse before analgesia is complete. Motor paralysis does not always accompany analgesia, particularly with weaker solutions.

Two areas of skin are usually not analgesic, one on the tip of the shoulder and the other on the medial aspect of the upper arm. If surgery is contemplated on the upper arm, an additional ring of infiltration is required in this area.

The axillary approach
The main advantage of this technique is that it avoids the potential though slight risk of pneumothorax and phrenic nerve paralysis involved in the supraclavicular method. The axillary approach is also somewhat simpler.

— The patient lies supine with the arm abducted to a right angle and the elbow flexed.
— Following shaving of axillary hair and the usual skin preparation, the anaesthetist palpates the axillary artery as high in the axilla as possible.
— An intradermal wheal is raised at the selected point, proximal to the lower border of the pectoralis major muscle.
— The needle is advanced through the wheal to one side of the axillary artery, which is 'guarded' by the palpating finger, until it penetrates the axillary fascial sheath. This is usually recognised as a definite click. Following a negative aspiration test 15–20 ml of lignocaine 1 per cent, with or without adrenaline 1 : 200 000, is injected. The needle is now withdrawn to the subcutaneous area and re-inserted on the other side of the axillary artery where the injection is repeated, again following a negative aspiration test.

Just as in the supraclavicular technique, a subcutaneous ring of injections in the upper arm may be required if analgesia is desired on the medial aspect of the upper arm.

Brachial plexus block by either of these two routes is especially suitable for surgical procedures on the forearm and hand. If a pneumatic tourniquet is used on the upper arm a 'dry field' can be provided which is ideal for tendon and peripheral nerve suturing.

PUDENDAL NERVE BLOCK

The majority of low forceps deliveries can be accomplished if this analgesic technique is employed. It is particularly suited for domiciliary obstetrical practice although at present widely used also in hospitals.

Anatomy. The pudendal nerve (S2, S3 and S4) leaves the pelvis via the greater sciatic foramen, passes across the ischial spine medial to the pudendal vessels and re-enters the pelvis via the lesser sciatic foramen. It then passes along the lateral wall of the ischio-rectal fossa in a sheath of fascia (Alcock's canal). This is the region where the nerve is most accessible for infiltration with analgesic solution.

Technique
— The ischial spine is palpated vaginally with one finger.
— The fingers of the other hand are inserted into the vagina with a 20 ml syringe, containing 1 per cent lignocaine with 1 : 200 000 adrenaline, held between the index and middle finger and lying in the palm of the hand.
— The needle is inserted laterally just beyond the ischial spine to a depth of about half an inch and following a negative aspiration test for blood, 10 ml of solution is injected. The injection is repeated on the other side.

SUBARACHNOID AND EPIDURAL ANALGESIA

It is convenient to consider the techniques of subarachnoid (spinal) analgesia and epidural analgesia together. In one method the drug is introduced into the cerebrospinal fluid in the subarachnoid space to produce motor, sensory and autonomic blockade by bathing the nerve roots as they leave the spinal cord. In the second method the local analgesic is introduced into the potential space immediately outside the dura mater and permeates the fatty areolar tissue there, contacting the nerves as they traverse the space (Figs 1.11 and 1.12). The actual site of action of the drug in epidural analgesia is not known precisely but it is probable that:

1. a true 'spinal' is produced by diffusion of the drug into the subarachnoid space through the dura mater, or
2. the local analgesic acts directly on the nerve roots ensheathed in dura in the epidural space, or
3. the spinal nerves are blocked in the intervertebral foramina beyond their dural sheaths.

Although epidural block is technically more difficult to perform than subarachnoid block it is preferred since there is a smaller chance of grave neurological sequelae. Spinal analgesia has in the past been complicated by frequent minor sequelae such as headache and by occasional disastrous complications such as paraplegia. These unpleasant results have followed apparently uneventful and meticulous procedures carried out by experts. Although neurological complications can follow epidural analgesia these are very rare and therefore most anaesthetists prefer this technique.

SPINAL ANALGESIA

Certain factors must be considered which influence the level of analgesia obtained when a drug is injected into the subarachnoid space.

The specific gravity of the solution. Cerebrospinal fluid has a specific gravity of 1001–1009 at body temperature and the local analgesic is classified according to whether it has the same specific gravity as cerebrospinal fluid (i.e. isobaric), or a greater specific gravity (i.e. hyperbaric), or a lower specific gravity (i.e. hypobaric). Hyperbaric and hypobaric solutions will travel up or down the subarachnoid space according to whether the patient is tilted head down or head up.

The posture of the patient. As mentioned above the posture of the patient during and for at least 15 minutes after injection, will influence the level of analgesia obtained. The sacral and dorsal spinal curves are sites at which the solution tends to 'pool' (Fig. 16.4).

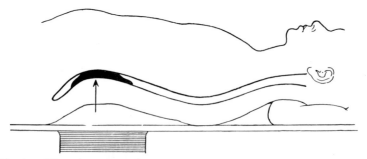

Fig. 16.4 When the patient roles over on to his back the height of the lumbar convexity corresponds to the level L2–3. The heavy solution now runs down both slopes. The part running into the sacral concavity is completely wasted as far as providing analgesia for abdominal surgery is concerned.

The site of injection. The higher the injection site the higher will be the resulting analgesia. Generally the interspaces between L2–3 and L3–4 are chosen for hyperbaric techniques.

The volume of solution injected. The height of analgesia is directly proportional to the volume of fluid injected.

The dose of drug injected. The greater the concentration of drug, the longer will its effect last.

The force and rate of injection. A rapid and forceful injection will result in the analgesic solution travelling further along the subarachnoid space from the site of injection.

As for most regional procedures light premedication is desirable. This allays the patient's natural anxiety and ensures a tranquil co-operative patient during the induction of analgesia.

It is important to remember that the analgesic solution will not be fixed for about 15 minutes following injection, and to avoid any movement which may result in the solution travelling too high

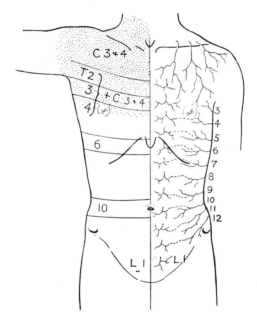

Fig. 16.5 Segmental levels of analgesia.

in the subarachnoid space. The progress of the analgesia can be determined by needle-prick of the skin of the abdominal wall, keeping in mind the segmental levels (Fig. 16.5).

During the interval following injection the anaesthetist should set up an intravenous infusion so that a ready route for drug administration is available. If a fall in arterial pressure is not desired a suitable dose of vasopressor, either intramuscularly or intravenously, should be given to the patient. Many patients are content to be drowsily awake during the subsequent surgery but their eyes should be gently blindfolded. A light general anaesthetic may be administered to others and this is usually the case with upper abdominal procedures.

EPIDURAL ANALGESIA

Subarachnoid analgesia is not popular nowadays and some of the reasons have already been mentioned. One other disadvantage is that where a high spinal block has been induced there is interference with ventilation because of the muscle paralysis involving the lower intercostals. This may necessitate assisting ventilation during the surgical procedure and any residual paralysis can be a danger in the early post-operative phase. Epidural analgesia, on the other hand, produces a differential block in that reflex muscle relaxation is produced without loss of motor power. This is accompanied by excellent analgesia and, if desired, autonomic block and hypotension. Although the technique is more difficult there is less chance of damage to the spinal cord. In addition, the epidural technique has many therapeutic applications outside of the operating theatre which make it a useful procedure.

The factors which influence the level of analgesia produced in an epidural block are:

The site of injection. The higher the injection the higher will be the analgesia. Usually the puncture is made in the lumbar region but for some purposes the upper thoracic interspaces are used. Here extreme care must be taken to avoid the spinal cord. The mid-thoracic region is dangerous and should be avoided.

The rate and force of injection. Just as in subarachnoid analgesia, a rapid forceful injection will result in the solution travelling further from the site of puncture and a higher level of analgesia will result.

The posture of the patient. A steep head-down tilt will result in the solution travelling higher and the level of analgesia will also be higher.

The volume of analgesic solution. Taller patients, having an epidural space of greater capacity, require a larger volume of solution if the same level of analgesia is to be obtained as in shorter patients.

The age of the patient. Elderly patients require a smaller volume of solution to produce any given level of analgesia.

Technique

The patient is premedicated with a barbiturate or an opiate as for spinal analgesia. The anaesthetist is gloved, gowned and masked and the patient's back is prepared as for any operative procedure. Two approaches are commonly used, one the caudal approach and the other the lumbar.

Caudal approach

— The patient lies face down on the operating table or trolley with legs apart and a pillow under the pelvis. The toes should be turned inwards. This position gives the best access to the sacral hiatus.

— The sacral hiatus, which results from the lack of fusion of the laminae of the 5th sacral vertebra and sometimes the 4th vertebra as well, is palpated. This is best done by sliding the finger upwards from the coccyx in the mid-line.

— An intradermal wheal is raised and a straight 22 gauge needle introduced at an angle of about 70–80° to the skin surface. This needle should not be more than 4.5 cm long to avoid penetration of the dural sac, which comes down to the level of the lower border of the 2nd sacral vertebra.

— When the needle penetrates the sacro-coccygeal membrane, and this is usually easy to recognise, it is depressed to an angle of 15–20° to the skin surface and it should then advance easily into the sacral canal. Two causes of failure to enter the sacral canal are:

1. The needle may be advanced superficial to the hiatus and the injection made subcutaneously with resulting swelling at the site of injection.
2. The needle may be inserted under the periosteum.

— Following a negative aspiration test for cerebrospinal fluid and blood, a test dose of 5 ml of 1.5 per cent lignocaine without adrenaline is injected.

— If no motor paralysis is evident after a period of 5 minutes, when the patient has been asked to move his toes, the rest of the injection is proceeded with. About 20 ml of 1.5 per cent lignocaine is required for operations on the anus such as excision of a fissure or haemorrhoids. The analgesia is complete in 10 minutes and lasts about one hour.

The anatomy of the caudal space is variable and the space may be loculated. This can result in unilateral analgesia.

Lumbar approach
To reach higher levels from the caudal approach larger volumes of analgesic would be required with a greater risk of toxic effects. The lumbar approach is therefore preferred for abdominal procedures. A special needle, the Tuohy needle, is used for a lumbar epidural analgesia (Fig. 16.6).

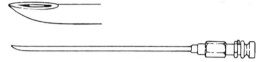

Fig. 16.6 The Tuohy needle. The trocar point and side opening can be seen.

A catheter introduced through the Tuohy needle, directed up or downwards by rotation of the needle, enables a continuous epidural analgesia to be administered. The catheter can be connected to a paediatric 'burette-type' intravenous set, thus ensuring absolute sterility.

This modification enables post-operative analgesia to be continued for hours or in some cases days and is a useful method in patients with severe respiratory disorders. The same technique, or the continuous caudal alternative, can be employed in labour particularly in cases of cervical dystocia. Other therapeutic indications for continuous epidural analgesia are the relief of pain in acute pancreatitis, for the relief of pain and autonomic blockade in peripheral vascular disease and arterial embolism in the legs.

Control of arterial pressure
The autonomic blockade which follows epidural analgesia results in hypotension. This can be of great advantage to the surgeon, providing a fairly bloodless field for major procedures such as Wertheim's hysterectomy. The blood pressure must not be permitted to fall below 60 mmHg in fit patients and any blood loss must be meticulously restored. Should hypotension be contra-indicated, a vasopressor such as methoxamine (2–10 mg) can be given intramuscularly or intravenously following completion of the epidural injection.

INTRAVENOUS REGIONAL ANALGESIA

This technique is at present enjoying a revival, and deservedly so, because of its simplicity and safety. First described by Bier in 1908 it is a useful method of analgesia for emergency surgery on the limbs. For operations on the arm and hand it is preferred by many to brachial plexus block which requires a greater degree of technical skill to accomplish and has occasional complications such as pneumothorax.

Method
A standard sphygmomanometer cuff, or a specially designed double cuff (Fig. 16.7), is placed round the patient's arm and the

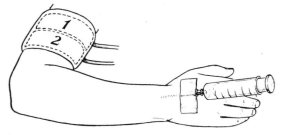

Fig. 16.7 Intravenous local analgesia. The upper cuff is inflated after the limb has been rendered bloodless. The injection is then made, the lower cuff inflated and finally the upper one deflated.

systolic blood pressure recorded. A needle or disposable plastic cannula is then introduced into a vein on the back of the hand, or forearm if the hand is involved in the injury. The limb is raised and emptied of blood by the application of an Esmarch bandage, applied from the hand proximally to the level of the blood pressure cuff which is then inflated to just above the systolic pressure. Forty ml (in a healthy 70 kg adult) of 0.5 per cent lignocaine without adrenaline is then injected into the needle or cannula for an arm (i.e. 200 mg lignocaine) or up to 100 ml for a leg (i.e. 500 mg of lignocaine). Paraesthesia usually develop during the injection and are immediately followed by profound analgesia and frequently complete muscle paralysis.

On completion of the surgical procedure power and sensation return to the limb within 5 to 10 minutes of release of the tourniquet.

Advantages
— A suitable technique for emergency procedures in patients not prepared for general anaesthesia.
— The technique is extremely simple and reliable.
— The risk of complications is much less than with brachial plexus block.

17

Techniques associated with anaesthesia

HYPOTHERMIA IN ANAESTHESIA

Moderate hypothermia, that is 28 to 32°C, is used clinically in two ways. It may be used in the *treatment of hyperpyrexia* when the body temperature increases to dangerous levels. This situation is met with following some head injuries and also following allergic reactions to drug therapy. The second clinical use of body cooling is in neurosurgery or less frequently nowadays in cardiovascular surgery where some operations can be performed during temporary occlusion of the circulation. The hypothermia protects the brain and other organs, for a limited period of time, from the effects of hypoxia. This is possible since the basal oxygen requirements of these tissues are reduced at low temperatures (Fig. 17.1).

Since the anaesthetist may require to induce hypothermia in the intensive care unit during the management of head injuries,

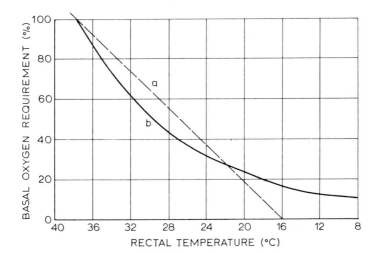

Fig. 17.1 The fall in oxygen requirement of the body with fall in temperature was thought to be a linear relationship (a), but is now known to be exponential (b).

and in the cardiothoracic theatre, some of the methods available are mentioned here.

Methods

Outside the operating theatre the technique of body surface cooling is the one commonly employed and this can be accomplished in many different ways. The following are some of the methods in use.

Ice-bags. The application of ice-bags to the patient's skin surface in the axillae, around the neck and in the groins is the simplest technique available. These sites are chosen because major arteries lie close to the surface and the blood is more readily cooled.

Immersion cooling. The patient can be immersed in a bath of water at a temperature of 15 to 18°C. The water is circulated over the body surface and this is a very effective cooling technique.

Cooling blanket. Special blankets containing a 'cooling coil' can be wrapped around the patient. A coolant like ethylene glycol or cold water is circulated through the coil.

Water spray cooling. Cold water is sprayed on to the skin surface and returned to a reservoir, from which it is pumped back to the spray again. This is really a variant of immersion cooling and is equally effective.

Surface air cooling. This technique requires a cooling cabinet through which cold air is blown by a fan and circulated over the patient's skin. This method permits of greater precision in attaining the desired degree of cooling.

Although any of the techniques described above can be used prior to cardiac surgery, the method generally preferred nowadays is blood-stream cooling. Here the patient is connected to a heart-lung machine combined with a heat exchanger which cools or warms the circulating blood as it is delivered to the patient from the oxygenator (Fig. 17.2).

Temperature measurement

The phrase 'body temperature' lacks precision and it is important to state the site at which any temperature reading is taken, for example oral, rectal, oesophageal or nasopharyngeal. During induced hypothermia, temperature gradients are set up throughout the body, since cooling of the tissues is not uniform. The body core is warmer than the skin surface and the brain may be at a different temperature from the liver.

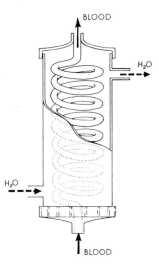

Fig. 17.2 A heat exchanger. The circulating blood passes through the coil and is cooled or heated by water in the surrounding jacket.

In order to control the cooling process properly, continuously recording thermometers capable of reading to low levels should be employed and not the usual mercury glass clinical type. Figures 10.3 and 10.4 show two types of thermometer which are suitable.

Control of the cooling process

The normal body reaction when exposed to cold is vasoconstriction and shivering. This protective mechanism must be overcome

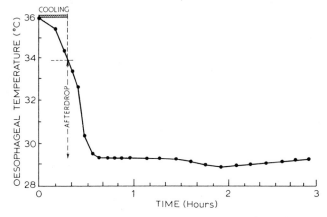

Fig. 17.3 A cooling chart showing the fall in temperature after active cooling has stopped—the after-drop.

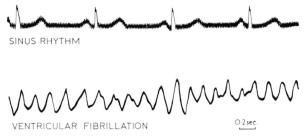

SINUS RHYTHM

VENTRICULAR FIBRILLATION   0·2 sec.

Fig. 17.4 Electrocardiograms of sinus rhythm and ventricular fibrillation.

if hypothermia is to be controlled. This is done by employing drugs which act centrally on the thermal nucleus in the hypothalamus and on the shivering centre in the thalamus. General anaesthetic agents and the phenothiazine drugs act in this way and assist the cooling process. Peripherally acting drugs, which prevent the muscle fibrillation and vasoconstriction found during shivering, may also be employed. The general anaesthetic agents again act in this way as do the curariform and ganglion blocking drugs.

When the active surface cooling process is stopped, the core temperature of the body continues to fall due to redistribution of heat in the body (Fig. 17.3). This 'after-drop' in temperature must be anticipated by stopping the cooling process in good time, otherwise the core temperature may fall below 28°C. Below this level cardiac arrhythmia is common and spontaneous ventricular fibrillation can occur (Fig. 17.4). If ventilation is not controlled, when the body temperature falls to the region of moderate hypothermia, ventilation becomes inadequate and the arterial carbon dioxide content rises with a resultant fall in pH. This respiratory acidosis occurs despite the reduction in carbon dioxide production that accompanies tissue cooling.

If hypothermia is to be a controlled process, it is evident that careful attention must be paid to the cardiovascular and respiratory state as well as to continual recording of the temperature at various sites in the body.

INDUCED HYPOTENSION IN ANAESTHESIA

For many surgical procedures a bloodless field is a great advantage. This is particularly true of plastic surgery and neurosurgery, but, since there are definite risks associated with the technique, generalised hypotension should not be used unless it is essential to the success of the surgical procedure. It should never be undertaken lightly but only after careful consideration of the patient's fitness for the procedure. Hypotension carries an increased risk where there is evidence of myocardial or cerebral ischaemia or where hepatic or renal function is abnormal.

Methods

High spinal analgesia. Sympathetic blockade with resulting hypotension can be produced by the subarachnoid injection of a local analgesic agent such as cinchocaine or lignocaine.

High epidural analgesia. Sympathetic blockade is produced by the injection of local analgesic solution in the epidural space.

Ganglion blocking drugs. Sympathetic blockade can be produced by the intravenous administration of drugs such as hexamethonium (Vegolysen) or trimetaphan (Arfonad). This is also obtained when curare and halothane are administered together.

Sodium nitroprusside. This drug has been reintroduced to clinical practice in recent years to produce a readily controlled hypotensive effect during anaesthesia, particularly for micro-surgery of the ear. It is used as an intravenous infusion of 0.002–0.01 per cent concentration, and produces its effect by direct action on the vessel walls independent of autonomic innervation. Duration of action is brief and tachyphylaxis does not occur. Overdose is to be avoided since metabolic acidosis and cardiovascular collapse can occur as a result of cyanide poisoning.

Anaesthetic technique

Whatever method is used to induce hypotension, the accompanying anaesthetic technique must be meticulous. Adequate oxygenation must be ensured throughout the procedure and respiration supported if at all inadequate. Although bleeding is reduced during surgery, accurate assessment of any blood loss and immediate replacement is essential, if normal blood pressure is to be successfully restored after the operation.

Hypotension can only be considered as 'controlled' if close attention is paid to the aforementioned points and if the arterial pressure is constantly and accurately measured. The systolic blood pressure should not be permitted to fall below 60–70 mmHg or renal damage with resulting post-operative renal failure may occur. The arterial pressure can be adjusted by altering the patient's posture, for example raising the lower limbs, or by giving a vasopressor drug such as methoxamine.

Post-operatively the patient must be nursed supine until the effects of the sympathetic blockade wear off. Arterial pressure readings should be made frequently, for the first hour or two post-operatively, until stable readings are obtained at the pre-operative values.

NEUROLEPTANALGESIA

Certain minor neurosurgical procedures and diagnostic procedures, such as cardiac catheterisation, may ideally be performed in patients who are sedated and free from pain, where muscular relaxation is not essential. The patient's co-operation is occasionally required during the procedure and therefore he or she should be capable of being aroused. This state of sedation and indifference to environment, combined with analgesia and the ability to co-operate when required, is known as neuroleptanalgesia. As yet, no one drug can produce these conditions, but various combinations have been tried with more or less success.

The technique is based on the combination of a neuroleptic drug, producing sedation or indifference to the environment, with a potent analgesic. The potent analgesics used, phenoperidine and fentanyl, are pethidine-like drugs and in large doses have similar disadvantages, namely respiratory depression, nausea and vomiting. The first of the neuroleptic drugs used, haloperidol, produced a fairly high incidence of side effects in the form of hallucinations and extra-pyramidal reactions. More recently dehydrobenzperidol (Droperidol) has been used but in larger doses it may also cause these unpleasant side effects. Evidence has also been produced to show that while some of the patients lie apparently calm and sedated they are experiencing hallucinations.

These side effects have so far limited the use of the technique. Nevertheless in this field research is continuing and exciting developments may be expected in the future.

ELECTRONARCOSIS

The question, 'Why is a drug an anaesthetic and how does it work?' is often asked. There is no doubt that the final answer is not yet available, since many diverse drugs can produce anaesthesia although apparently acting in quite different ways. In addition, various physical means of producing insensibility and freedom from pain are known and, for many years, it has been apparent that electrical currents passed through the brain can produce unconsciousness and freedom from pain for short intervals, for example during electroconvulsive therapy. This approach has enjoyed a revival recently and anaesthesia or electronarcosis produced in this way is being used in some centres.

The advantages of this technique are obvious in that, since no drug is administered, there is no concern about liver.function and renal function with regard to drug elimination. Respiratory and cardiovascular depression are minimal and post-operative recovery is rapid and free from drug 'hangover'. Although the method is not yet widely accepted, it is attractive enough to warrant further trial and investigation.

ACUPUNCTURE

This technique, used for centuries by Chinese physicians in treatment of a wide variety of diseases and relief of pain, is at present being extensively studied. It consists of the insertion of needles at selected points on lines or meridia which can be determined by reference to charts. The needles are then either rotated or electrically stimulated for a varying length of time. The acupuncture sites bear no anatomical relation to the areas of pain relief and the method defies explanation in Western physiological terms. It appears to produce results in China far in excess of those obtained elsewhere, certainly in regard to production of anaesthesia, and it may be that hypnotic suggestion and acceptance—as with many other therapeutic measures—are largely responsible.

At present considerable interest is being expressed in the use of this method and further information on the place of the technique in anaesthesia is awaited.

18

The anaesthetist in consultation

By virtue of his special knowledge of the management of respiratory problems in the operating theatre and his familiarity with a wide range of drugs and their antidotes, the anaesthetist has a role to play outside the traditional confines of the operating theatre. His advice and technical assistance may be required in the management of therapeutic problems which fall broadly into two groups.

The first group is where *intractable pain* is a problem, for example in terminal carcinoma; tic douloureux, etc. Here he can often help, because of his familiarity with the techniques of local analgesia. The injection of solutions of local analgesic into the epidural or subarachnoid spaces can also be used to relieve severe pain and, in terminal carcinoma of the pelvic organs, a *permanent block* can be performed by injecting a solution of *phenol* or *alcohol* into the extradural space, destroying all pain-carrying fibres from the affected area. In some hospitals pain clinics have been established under the general supervision of the anaesthetic department.

The second group of problems with which the anaesthetist has to deal are *respiratory in origin*. The anaesthetist is using techniques involving the control of respiration daily and is constantly measuring and assessing respiratory function. These respiratory problems may arise pre-operatively or post-operatively or may be unassociated with any surgical problem, for example polyneuritis or severe myasthenia gravis.

The common causes of surgical respiratory problems fall readily into five groups.

Pre-existing lung disease
Pre-existing lung disease, unrecognised pre-operatively, is one of the commonest causes of post-operative respiratory failure. Patients with chronic airways disease usually suffer from acute exacerbation of their disease during the winter months and are

always on the verge of lung failure. Even minor surgery, requiring general anaesthesia, can have a similar effect and result in acute respiratory failure. It is very important that such patients should, whenever possible, have pulmonary function tests and blood-gas analyses performed pre-operatively in order to assess the severity of their disease and thus the advisability of surgery. If operation is essential, the particular anaesthetic technique best suited to them can be chosen. When elective surgery is contemplated there is time for full investigation and to institute a prophylactic regime of antibiotics, broncho-dilator drugs, postural drainage and physiotherapy. A tracheostomy may be indicated. General anaesthesia may be contra-indicated and many procedures can be done under epidural or regional analgesia instead.

There are two other types of patient who may be conveniently discussed here. The first is the grossly obese patient with respiratory embarrassment. Here the lungs themselves may be normal but the patient suffers from dyspnoea on exertion, due to the increased oxygen demands resulting from the effort of maintaining mobility. Further disablement results from poor muscle tone in the respiratory musculature and splinting of the diaphragm by the abdominal contents. These patients must be dieted rigorously pre-operatively, and physiotherapy can be of assistance.

The second type of case is the patient suffering from constrictive disease of the thorax, for example ankylosing spondylitis, where again the lungs may be normal but the respiratory excursion of the thorax severely limited. Regional or epidural analgesia is again preferred here for intra-abdominal surgery.

The quick return of an active cough reflex post-operatively is particularly important in all patients with pre-existing lung disease, in order that secretions may not accumulate in the bronchi giving rise to the typical post-operative chest, such as atelectasis or pulmonary collapse and pneumonia (Fig. 18.1).

Traumatic conditions
Patients with multiple injuries may first present as acute respiratory problems. For instance, a severe facio-maxillary injury often has upper airway obstruction and is in imminent danger of asphyxiating unless a clear airway is secured before surgery is contemplated. In an emergency, an endotracheal tube may be introduced, and oxygen, with perhaps assistance to ventilation given. A tracheostomy may then be performed if there is doubt about maintenance of the airway, after corrective surgery is completed.

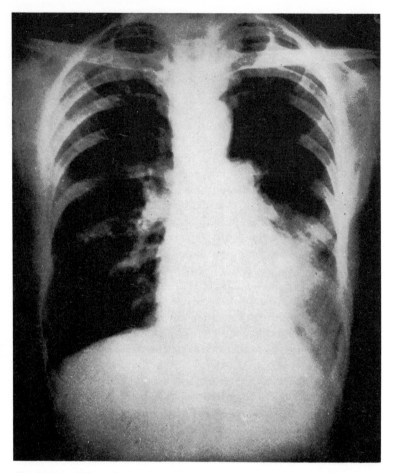

Fig. 18.1 A radiograph showing collapse of the lower lobe of the left lung.

Patients with severe head injuries, in deep coma, are in grave danger of obstruction of the airway either from the tongue falling back against the posterior pharyngeal wall or by inhalation of regurgitated gastric contents while the cough reflex is depressed. At an early stage the airway should be secured by means of an endotracheal tube or tracheostomy, and the stomach emptied. Damage to the vital centres, including the respiratory centre, may cause inadequate respiration or occasionally apnoea may ensue. This is an indication for assistance to ventilation either by hand or by a mechanical ventilator.

Trauma to the chest wall—'crushed chest' or 'stove-in-chest'— is worthy of special mention. This high-velocity impact injury is becoming increasingly common in car accidents. As a result of this injury a segment of the thoracic wall, most frequently lateral but occasionally anterior, is floating free due to rib fractures anteriorly and posteriorly (Fig. 18.2). The underlying lung is also contused and there may be a pneumothorax or haemopneumothorax. In the worst examples of this the patient presents in acute respiratory failure with grave hypoxia and hypercarbia.

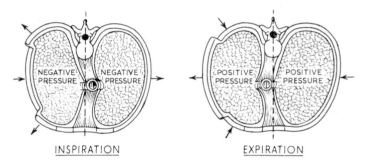

Fig. 18.2 The 'crushed-chest' injury. The paradoxical movement of the damaged chest wall and the movement of the mediastinum during respiration can be seen.

Four things happen when such a patient tries to breathe spontaneously:
1. On inspiration the thoracic cage expands but the floating segment is sucked in. On expiration the thorax retracts and the floating segment is pushed out.
2. Mediastinal shift occurs, leading to a reduction in central venous return and consequent reduction in cardiac output and heart failure.
3. Interpulmonary 'shunting' of gas occurs so that, on inspiration, the fresh gas entering the intact lung is diluted with gas, low in oxygen but high in carbon dioxide, from the damaged side. On expiration some of the gases from the intact lung enter the damaged side instead of being vented to atmosphere.
4. The alveoli in the damaged lung are unable to take part in normal ventilation resulting in hypoxia and hypercarbia. This latter factor is probably the most important single cause of respiratory failure in these patients.

It is obvious that this state of acute respiratory failure must be treated quickly and adequately before any surgery is embarked upon. Immediate endotracheal intubation with IPPV and oxygen and insertion of a water-sealed drain on the damaged side (in case of tension pneumothorax and to drain the haemothorax) is essential. Later a tracheostomy may be performed, as many of these patients require prolonged mechanical assistance to ventilation. IPPV with oxygen reverses most of the ill-effects of the crushed chest immediately, for example paradoxical respiration and shunting of gas in the lungs, and an immediate clinical improvement is usually obvious. In very few of these cases of crushed chest injury is surgery indicated, such as wiring ribs or applying external traction. In most cases IPPV and the measures described are sufficient by themselves.

Surgery on lungs and airway, etc.

It is obvious that, in a patient already suffering from lung disease, removal of diseased lung, with inevitably some normal lung tissue as well, as in lobectomy and pneumonectomy, may result in respiratory failure. The effect of removal of one or other lung in such a patient can often be predicted pre-operatively by differential bronchospirometry. Here lung function studies can be carried out on each lung separately and the result of removal of one or other lung predicted.

Surgery in the neck, for example thyroidectomy, can present some problems so far as respiratory function is concerned. In malignant disease of the thyroid or in thyroiditis, for example Hashimoto's disease, the gland may obstruct the underlying airway. This results in narrowing of the airway—'scabbard trachea'—and there may be a marked respiratory stridor. Tracheostomy under local analgesia before the thyroidectomy is occasionally necessary, and cases occur where a tracheostomy is required post-operatively, due to complete respiratory obstruction resulting from damage to the recurrent laryngeal nerves.

Abnormal response to drugs and drug overdose

An interesting group of patients who come to surgery are those suffering from a variety of relatively rare conditions which may have been diagnosed before surgery for some other coincident disease, for example myasthenia gravis, porphyria and a genetically transmitted condition in which a plasma enzyme, pseudocholinesterase, is deficient.

Patients with myasthenia gravis are abnormally sensitive to the competitive or non-depolarising muscle relaxants commonly used during anaesthesia. A prolonged post-operative respiratory muscle paralysis results, requiring mechanical assistance to ventilation until the drug effect wears off.

In porphyric patients, the use of barbiturates for induction of anaesthesia can result in an acute axacerbation of the condition with respiratory muscle paralysis post-operatively, and again prolonged mechanical assistance to ventilation will be required.

Another relaxant drug commonly used during anaesthesia is suxamethonium, which normally has a short action, being destroyed by an enzyme called pseudocholinesterase occurring in

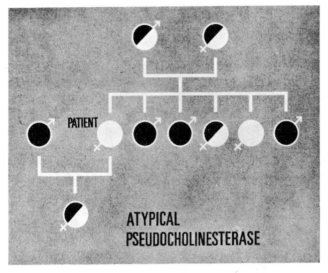

Fig. 18.3 Family tree demonstrating the genetic linkage of the condition of atypical pseudocholinesterase. One sister of the patient was also homozygous for the condition while other relatives were heterozygous or normal.

normal plasma. One group of patients have either an abnormally low pseudocholinesterase level or a normal amount of a different type of pseudocholinesterase which does not hydrolyse suxamethonium.

A typical family tree demonstrating the genetic aspect of this condition is illustrated (Fig. 18.3). Some patients are heterozygous for the condition and some homozygous.

The anaesthetist is required to assist all too often nowadays in the resuscitation of victims of drug overdosage. The barbiturates are commonly the drugs taken, although phenothiazines, tranquillisers, aspirin and occasionally opiates are responsible for the symptoms. In mild cases, the only treatment required, in addition to any specific antidote, is the routine posturing of the patient in the comparatively safe tonsillar position to avoid aspiration of regurgitated stomach contents. A further measure is intubation of the stomach and gastric lavage, not only in an attempt to recover any drug which may not yet have been absorbed but also to empty the stomach and again obviate regurgitation of its contents. A word of warning is in order here since it is all too easy, in an unconscious patient, to intubate the lungs and drown the patient during the gastric lavage. It is advisable, wherever possible, to carry out endo-tracheal intubation with a cuffed tube prior to the attempt at lavage. This also enables endotracheal suction to be carried out and guarantees an unobstructed airway during the patient's re-covery.

In more severe cases, the clinical state of the patient may war-rant other, more active, measures. Severe respiratory depression must be treated by assisted ventilation. This is done in the usual way via a cuffed endotracheal tube delivering oxygen either manu-ally or by a mechanical ventilator. Forced diuresis or dialysis with the artificial kidney may be employed in suitable cases but close attention must always be paid to the patient's respiratory and car-diovascular condition, throughout the period of drug action. Such energetic measures are time-consuming and require the services of skilled nursing and medical personnel, and an intensive care unit is the ideal place to treat those severely ill patients.

Other diseases presenting respiratory problems
The anaesthetist may be required to assist in the treatment of cer-tain medical conditions where interference with normal respira-tion is a feature. The disturbance of respiratory function may be a direct result of the disease, as in poliomyelitis, polyneuritis or myasthenia gravis, where weakness and paralysis of the respiratory musculature exists. On the other hand, in diseases such as tetanus or status epilepticus, there may be temporary interference with respiration during the convulsions.

Mechanical assistance to ventilation may be required for long periods where there is respiratory paralysis, and usually these patients have had a tracheostomy performed. The management of such cases is well understood and can be undertaken in the in-tensive care unit or the respiratory unit of an infectious diseases hospital. Control of the convulsions of severe tetanus or status epi-lepticus can be accomplished by administering muscle relaxants and, in this way, the management of the patient becomes similar to that of the paralysed patient with poliomyelitis. A preliminary tracheostomy is usually necessary and the airway is thus safe-guarded from danger of obstruction, and oxygenation and carbon dioxide elimination assured. This method of treatment avoids the dangers of acute hypoxic incidents which can result in cerebral damage or death in severe tetanus and status epilepticus. Specific therapy for the particular condition must be simultaneously carried out. In the case of tetanus this is the administration of anti-biotics and anti-tetanic serum, and in the case of status epilepticus treatment with diazepam, sodium phenobarbitone or phenytoin (Epanutin). Controlled ventilation is continued until convulsions cease and thereafter normal spontaneous respiration is permitted.

It can be seen that the anaesthetist can be of assistance to his surgical and medical colleagues in many widely differing circum-stances.

19

Mishaps and their medico-legal aspects

Alex C. Forrester, M.B., Ch.B., F.R.C.S.(G.), F.F.A.R.C.S.
Emeritus Professor of Anaesthesia, University of Glasgow

In the practice of anaesthesia, resuscitation and intensive care, many mishaps may overtake a doctor unless he is constantly on the alert. While a number of these unfortunate occurrences lie within the province of the specialist anaesthetist, some may be encountered by a student or resident, and are included in this chapter to illustrate the hazards which may face them. At the present time, there is an increasing tendency for patients to seek redress at law for any untoward incident which may occur, and it is essential to take adequate precautions when undertaking any procedure known to be associated with complications. A doctor cannot be held to be negligent if he has exercised a reasonable degree of skill and care, no matter what accident has occurred. In the same way, the occurrence of a well-recognised hazard does not of itself constitute negligence.

The mishaps to be considered fall conveniently into groups.

Mishaps associated with injections

Intra-arterial thiopentone.
Mention has been made in an earlier chapter (p. 84) of the effects of injecting thiopentone into the perivenous tissues or into an artery.

The following case histories illustrate what may happen when an intra-arterial injection of thiopentone is given.

Case 1. A male patient, aged 38, suffering from hypotension and shock was being anaesthetised. After the usual precautions had been taken, 2 ml of 5 per cent thiopentone were injected into a vessel in the medial antecubital fossa. After a pause, during which no pain was experienced, a further 2 ml were injected. Only then did the patient complain of pain. This was localised to the site of injection and passed off within a minute. Although a small flushed spot developed over the vessel, no other abnormality was noticed and anaesthesia was induced. It was considered that only a slight perivenous leakage had occurred and the surgeon proceeded with the operation. Twenty minutes later, patchy cyanosis was noted in the left forearm and the full picture of an arterial occlusion developed over the next sixteen hours. In spite of all methods of treatment, recognised at the time, including intra-arterial tolazoline and procaine, brachial plexus and stellate ganglion block, heparinisation and arteriotomy, a below-elbow amputation was necessary.

This case emphasises the increased risk of accidental intra-arterial injection of thiopentone in shocked patients. With impaired circulation, pulsation will be diminished and the onset of pain may be delayed.

Case 2. A healthy woman, aged 32, for ligation of varicose veins was given 1.5 ml of 5 per cent thiopentone into a vessel in the back of the hand. Agonising, burning pain was experienced in the wrist and hand, accompanied by intense blanching of the ulnar two-thirds of the dorsum of the hand and proximal dorsal surfaces of the medial two fingers. Following intra- and peri-arterial procaine, 5 ml of 1 per cent by each route, recovery occurred within ten minutes, the intense blanching being followed by reactive hyperaemia.

Although choosing an injection site on the back of the hand does not obviate the risk of intra-arterial injection, tissue necrosis is less likely to occur as there is an extensive collateral circulation in this area. In the unlikely event of an end artery being entered, at worst only a finger might be lost. By avoiding the medial antecubital fossa, damage to the median nerve is also eliminated.

In addition to avoiding the antecubital fossa one should as a routine ask if the patient feels pain locally or distal to the injection site after injection of 1–2 ml of solution. In 1962 an anaesthetist was found negligent where he had failed to ask this question and only won his appeal because no pain had been felt.

The routine use of 2.5 per cent solution of thiopentone is also highly desirable. Experimentally, it has been shown that, using the same total dose of thiopentone intra-arterial injection of 10 per cent solution, invariably produces gangrene, 5 per cent almost invariably so while 2.5 per cent solution never does. Clinically only one case of gangrene has been reported following intra-arterial injection of 2.5 per cent thiopentone.

At one time the use of 2.5 per cent solution was decried because the pH of the 5 per cent and 2.5 per cent solutions are similar— both over 10, and it it was thought that the alkalinity of the solution which caused arterial spasm was responsible for the gangrene which followed.

This has now been disproved and the thiopentone itself is responsible by causing intimal damage and subsequent thrombosis.

Methohexitone 1 per cent propanidid 5 per cent and Althesin are less irritant even than 2.5 per cent thiopentone.

The methods of treatment of this accident are given in Chapter 9 (p. 110).

Indirect arterial damage
Apart from damage to an artery by injecting an irritant drug into it, it is possible to cause damage to the artery by injecting a drug close to it.

In one case, hydroxydione was injected into a large vein in the antecubital fossa, and severe spasm of the brachial artery followed, resulting in amputation of the arm. Examination of the limb revealed no direct arterial damage or clotting and the spasm was considered to be due to perivenous leakage of the hydroxydione. In a second patient, injection of hydroxydione into an intravenous infusion at the wrist caused transient spasm of the radial artery.

It is also possible to deposit an irritant solution close to an artery by intramuscular injection, and gangrene of the arm has been reported following intramuscular injection of chlorpormazine in the upper arm close to the brachial artery.

Damage to the median nerve
In the antecubital fossa the median nerve lies close to the median cubital vein (Fig. 19.1), and is at risk if an injection is made in this area.

The following case illustrates this danger.

Case 3. A woman of 40 years was admitted for repair of a hernia. A needle, with a syringe attached, containing 10 ml of thiopentone 5 per cent was

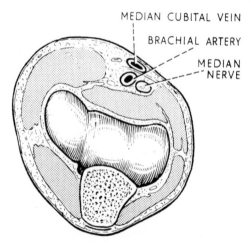

Fig. 19.1 A section of the antecubital fossa showing the proximity of the brachial artery and median nerve to the median cubital vein.

inserted into an antecubital vein in the left arm and venous blood aspirated. After one ml was injected the patient complained of some pain at the site of injection and a tingling sensation and numbness of the fingers of the hand. The needle was withdrawn and anaesthesia induced with nitrous oxide and oxygen.

On regaining consciousness the patient experienced loss of sensation in the fingers and palm accompanied by weakness in her hand; a median nerve palsy had resulted. Although she had a repair of the damaged nerve she was left with permanently defective sensation in her thumb and fingers and difficulty in handling objects with her left hand.

The close proximity of the median nerve to the antecubital vein was pointed out by Pask and Robson in 1954. They were of the opinion that slight movement of the patient's arm might advance a needle from the vein to the nerve, and it follows that it is wiser to make injections in some other region.

Local injection of vasoconstrictors
The danger of injecting solutions containing adrenaline in the vicinity of an end artery has been stressed (p. 209), particularly in the presence of local infection. The oxygen demand of the tissues is increased and when the blood supply is reduced gangrene may result. Figure 19.2 shows gangrene of a thumb following a ring block using procaine with 1 : 30 000 adrenaline.

Systemic use of vasoconstrictors
Noradrenaline infusions are used in patients with severe hypotension arising from different causes. Many of these patients are in

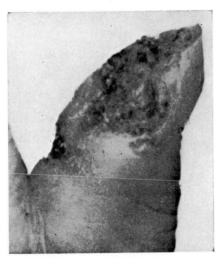

Fig. 19.2 Gangrene resulting from injection of local analgesic solution containing adrenaline at the base of the thumb.

a critical condition and often the infusion is made through a drip, set up for other purposes, often in the hand or arm. The danger of using such a peripheral vein for these vasoconstrictors is shown in Figures 19.3 and 19.4. Here gangrene of the hand and forearm

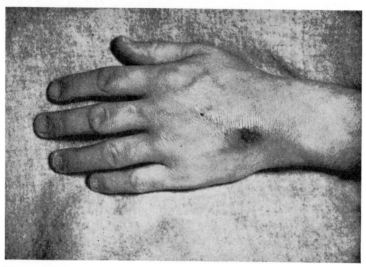

Fig. 19.3 Skin necrosis following noradrenaline infusion into a vein on the dorsum of the hand.

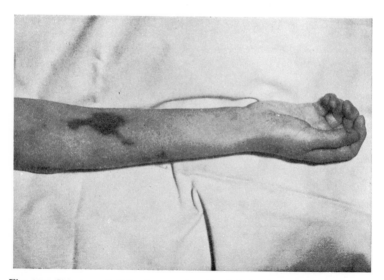

Fig. 19.4 Skin necrosis following noradrenaline infusion into a vein in the forearm.

are shown where these areas have been used. This is caused by the intense local vasoconstriction which is caused by the noradrenaline and, when such a drug is administered, a polythene cannula should be inserted until its tip lies within a large free running vein. This will cause rapid dilution of the drug.

If the skin overlying the vein shows colour changes other than slight blanching, the infusion should be stopped at once. Procaine or tolazoline injected into the vein may minimise the vasoconstriction. Nevertheless, two cases have been reported where polythene tubes were inserted 15 and 8 inches respectively into a large vein. Ulcers occurred in both cases at the tips of the cannulae. It may be that these infusions should be administered into the vena cava. Should ischaemia of the skin occur, the use of piperoxamine hydrochloride has been suggested to counteract this, 5 mg in 20 ml saline being injected around the vein.

The disappearing catheter

The advantage of placing a polythene catheter in a vein without exposing and tying off the vein is considerable. One method of doing this is to insert a metal needle through which a polythene cannula is passed. This technique has however brought its own hazards and if the polythene catheter is withdrawn through the needle it may be cut on the sharp edge and a portion of catheter

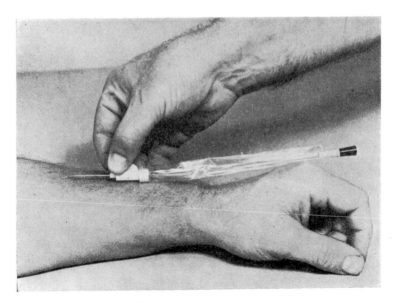

Fig. 19.5 The Deseret E–Z catheter unit.

left lying free in the vein. This in turn may migrate towards the heart with serious consequences. This type of set has now been modified. A new approach is that shown in Figure 19.5 where the needle is inside the plastic catheter and after insertion is withdrawn by means of a stilette.

The wrong solution

Great care must be taken to ensure that the solution to be injected, in whatever site, is that which it is intended to use. If the solution comes from a bottle or ampoule, check it with the label or engraving on the ampoule. Do not use fluid from an unlabelled ampoule or bottle either direct or to mix with powder or crystals. This habit has resulted in procaine crystals being mixed with an unlabelled solution which was in fact 1 : 1500 cinchocaine. Another accident is illustrated by Case 4.

Case 4. A brachial plexus block was being performed to remove a piece of metal from the hand. The house surgeon put surgical spirit in one galley pot for cleansing the skin while the anaesthetist prepared lignocaine 2 per cent in a similar galley pot. Unfortunately, the skin was cleaned with the lignocaine and the spirit was used for injection.

After 9 ml had been injected the mistake was noticed. The anaesthetist diluted the spirit by injecting into the same area a large quantity of very dilute lignocaine. Analgesia was complete and the foreign body was removed. About two days later, it was apparent that damage had been done to the brachial plexus. The patient was left with considerable disability including stiffness of the joints with muscular weakness and disturbed sensation.

Mishaps due to respiratory obstruction

Endotracheal anaesthesia is frequently employed to ensure a free airway. The use of an endotracheal tube does not, however, guarantee that respiratory obstruction will not take place. It has been shown that under certain circumstances tubes may kink, become blocked or dislodged. A death has occurred following herniation of the cuff over the end of an endotracheal tube (Fig. 19.6).

Case 5. A lady of 38 years was undergoing an operation for excision of a cervical rib. A cuffed endotracheal tube was passed and the patient was then turned into the prone position. Spontaneous respiration was satisfactory for half an hour, then movement of the reservoir bag ceased. The cause of the respiratory obstruction was later found to be herniation of the cuff over the end of the tube. This may have been caused by a steady traction on the tube due to the weight of the corrugated tubing and connections. The patient died ten days later from the results of cerebral hypoxia.

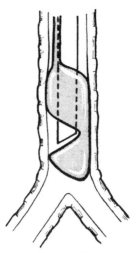

Fig. 19.6 A diagram illustrating the herniation of the cuff over the end of an endotracheal tube, resulting in respiratory obstruction.

Case 6. A somewhat similar accident occurred when using a latex armoured tube. The herniation developed internally, obstructing the lumen completely when the cuff was fully inflated. Fortunately, however, in this case the anaesthetist deflated the cuff and the obstruction was immediately relieved.

The use of disposable plastic endotracheal tubes may be the answer to this problem.

Probably the most common mishap in endotracheal anaesthesia is accidental intubation of the right main bronchus due to the use of too long an endotracheal tube.

Case 7. Figure 19.7 shows a tube in the right bronchus with total collapse of the left lung. The bifurcation of the trachea is never lower than the upper border of the 5th thoracic vertebra. The tube here extends to at least the lower border of the 5th vertebra. There is also narrowing of the rib spaces, and mediastinal shift to the collapsed side.

In this case the accident was noticed only at the completion of the operation, when breathing became inadequate. Blood gas examination revealed a Pa_{CO_2} of 13.6 kPa. Following bronchoscopy, suction and assisted ventilation for about two hours, the patient made a complete recovery.

While the emphasis has here been placed on endotracheal tubes, the residents in an intensive care unit should always be aware of the dangers attendant on the displacement of a tracheostomy tube, or its obstruction by inspissated mucus.

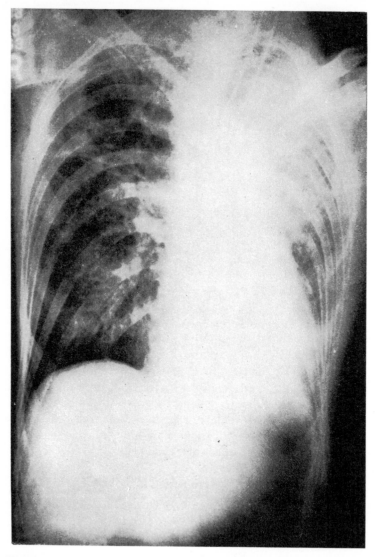

Fig. 19.7 A radiogram showing an endotracheal tube in the right main bronchus and collapse of the left lung.

Vomiting during anaesthesia

Despite the attention which has been focused on the problem, deaths from inhalation of vomitus still occur. A recent death resulted from lack of liaison between the anaesthetist, surgeon and nursing staff.

Case 8. A patient was admitted to hospital for possible Caesarean section. Two hours later she was given a full meal, unknown to the anaesthetist and surgeon. One hour after this, anaesthesia was induced with thiopentone. In the course of induction the patient vomited and, despite all efforts, died shortly afterwards from asphyxia.

This case gave rise to litigation and emphasises the need for full co-operation between nursing and medical staff (Chapter 4).

Peripheral nerve injuries

Although spontaneous nerve injuries do occur, damage usually follows the use of unsuitable tourniquets or posture. Recently a patient suffered a median and radial nerve palsy following the use of an Esmarch bandage on the upper arm. It would appear wise in applying tourniquets to follow the recommendations described below:

— In the upper arm, a pneumatic cuff should be routinely employed.
— In the lower limb, if an Esmarch bandage is used, it should be applied only in the mid-thigh and then only over a towel.
— The maximum period of application should not be longer than two hours.
— Precautions should be instituted which will guarantee the removal of the tourniquet at the end of the operation, for example tourniquet tied to the table.

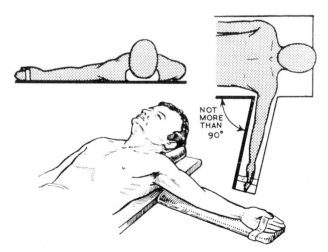

NOT MORE THAN 90°

Fig. 19.8 The correct position of the arm board is shown.

The other form of nerve injury associated with operation and anaesthesia is damage to the brachial plexus by incorrect positioning of the arms during infusion (the correct position is shown in Figure 19.8), or by the incorrect use of shoulder rests. This latter difficulty can be overcome by use of non-slip corrugated mattresses (Fig. 19.9).

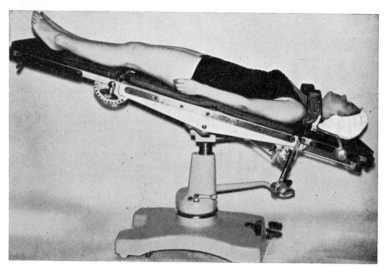

Fig. 19.9 The Trendelenburg position: the non-slip mattress shown here is of itself sufficient to prevent the patient sliding off the table. The shoulder rests, shown in use here, are essential if a plain mattress is used, but these must be positioned in such a way that damage to the brachial plexus is avoided.

These mishaps are associated with techniques which are in widespread use and are often life-saving. Their occurrence should not detract from the techniques, but rather ensure scrupulous care in their application.

Explosions

While explosions in the operating theatre are less common now than when ethers were more widely used, the attention of all persons working in the anaesthetic room and operating theatre should be drawn to the potential hazards (see Warning Notice, p. 249).

Scottish Home and Health Department

Fires and explosions in operating theatres and anaesthetic rooms

WARNING NOTICE

Flammable anaesthetic agents such as ether, cyclopropane and ethyl chloride when mixed with air, oxygen or nitrous oxide may form explosive mixtures, and the ignition of such anaesthetic vapours has resulted in explosions which have been attended by serious consequences. The chief causes of such ignitions are:

(a) Electrostatic spark discharge. This is more likely to occur during dry atmospheric conditions and in particular during the early part of a session when conditions tend to be driest.

(b) Sparking at electrical contacts, diathermy electrodes, etc.

(c) Use of apparatus incorporating hot surfaces, for example cautery, electric heaters, overheated lamps.

(d) Gas or spirit burners.

Whenever an explosive mixture is in use the surgeon and the theatre sister should be aware of the fact.

PRECAUTIONS AND RECOMMENDATIONS

1. Anti-static precautions

The best means of reducing electrostatic risks is to eliminate the use of materials which readily electrify in normal use. *The chief sources of static electricity are insulating rubber, plastics, wool, nylon.* Experience suggests that non-conducting rubber breathing equipment on anaesthetic apparatus constitutes the greatest risk. Materials which are anti-static for practical purposes are available, for example, anti-static rubber, anti-static rubber-proofed fabrics, linen, cotton and viscose, and should be used wherever possible instead of the electrostatic materials.

Recommended anti-static precautionary measures:
(a) *Rubberised anaesthetic breathing equipment and rubber tubing* used with suction apparatus, etc., should have permanent anti-static properties.

(b) *Operating tables, anaesthetic apparatus, patients' and other trolleys, stools, etc.*, should have metal or anti-static rubber-tyred castors or feet. The metal work of anaesthetic and other apparatus should be electrically continuous and top surfaces and shelves should be free from paint or other insulating finish.

(c) *Rubber pads* on operating tables, trolleys or stools should have permanent anti-static properties or be completely enclosed in an anti-static fabric, for example cotton, linen or viscose rayon.

(d) *All persöns entering an anaesthetising location should wear anti-static footwear and a reasonable close-fitting outer garment of an anti-static fabric.* Anti-static rubber-soled footwear is considered preferable. Other types should be enclosed in overboots of an anti-static fabric, for example cotton or linen.

(e) *Floors should have suitable permanent anti-static properties,* for example anti-static quality terrazzo, terrazzo tile, PVC or ceramic tile floors.

2. Electrical apparatus

(a) *Switch contacts* and other parts of apparatus capable of producing an incendive spark should be housed in a gas-tight enclosure or spaced at least 4 feet horizontally from any anaesthetic apparatus.

(b) The maximum *voltage* of circuits used for energising endoscopes, etc., should be as *low* as is practicable and not appreciably higher than the rated voltage of the lamps. The provision of a special current limiting resistance in the circuit will greatly reduce the spark and overheating risks. *Dry-cell batteries* are safer than mains transformers for operating endoscopes.

(c) *Electrically operated suction apparatus* should have no sparking contacts which are open to atmosphere, and the exhaust outlet from the pump should terminate outside any enclosure housing the apparatus.

(d) From the electrical safety aspect *surgical tools* operated by means of compressed air are considered preferable to electrically operated tools, because of the inherent spark and electric shock risks associated with the latter.

(e) Flexible *cables* should be free from joints, frequently inspected and renewed when damaged or showing signs of deterioration.

(f) The risks associated with *diathermy and cautery apparatus* are obvious. Before these are used following the administration of flammable anaesthetics a non-flammable gas should be passed through the breathing circuit until no explosive residue remains either in the apparatus or in the patient's lungs. The ether bottle and cyclopropane cylinder should be removed. It is not sufficient to rely on turning these taps off as they might not be gas-tight.

3. Open flames and heated surfaces

Apparatus incorporating open flame burners or heated surfaces which may operate at temperatures of 350°F or more can constitute an ignition risk if located within 20 feet of an anaesthetising position. Doors between the anaesthetising position and the ignition risk should not be regarded as a reliable safeguard, as they may be left open.

NOTES—Spirits lotions, etc. It should be noted that the use of spirit, spirit lotions and other flammable solutions which are frequently employed for cleansing the patient's skin, etc., involves dangers similar to those mentioned above. Additional information on the risks referred to above, together with recommended precautions against associated risks, are contained in 'Report of a Working Party on Anaesthetic Explosions' and Hospital Technical Memoranda Nos. 1 and 2 (HMSO).

Further safety precautions

In addition, there must be no smoking in the anaesthetic room or theatre precincts and *all theatre personnel* must be aware when an explosive mixture is in use. In any location where oxygen is being administered the precautions outlined in the warning notice should be observed. This applies equally to areas in general wards.

APPENDIX

SI units

The International System of Units (Système International, SI) was adopted in 1960 by the General Conference of Weights and Measures as a logical, coherent system based on seven fundamental units: metre, kilogram, second, ampere, kelvin, candela and mole.

The system has been adopted generally by international scientific bodies, including the International Federation of Clinical Chemistry (IFCC) and the Section of Clinical Chemistry of the International Union of Pure and Applied Chemistry (IUPAC).

All measurements are expressed in the basic units or in units derived from them. The seven basic units, and some of the derived units relevant to medicine with standard abbreviations are:

Physical quantiy	Name of SI Unit	Symbol
length	metre	m
mass	kilogram	kg
time	second	s
electric current	ampere	A
temperature	kelvin	K
luminous intensity	candela	cd
amount of substance	mole	mol
energy	joule	J
force	newton	N
power	watt	W
pressure	pascal	Pa

Prefixes to indicate fractions or multiples of the basic or derived units have also been defined.

Prefixes for SI units

Factor	Name	Symbol	Factor	Name	Symbol
10^{18}	Exa-	E	10^{18}	Atto-	a
10^{15}	Peta-	P	10^{15}	Femto-	f
10^{12}	Tera-	T	10^{12}	Pico-	p
10^{9}	Giga-	G	10^{9}	Nano-	n
10^{6}	Mega-	M	10^{6}	Micro-	μ
10^{3}	Kilo-	k	10^{3}	Milli-	m
10^{2}	Hecto-	h	10^{2}	Centi-	c
10	Deca-	da	10^{1}	Deci-	d

Blood chemistry. Units and conversion factors

Measurement	SI unit	Old unit	Conversion factors	
			Old to SI (exact)	SI to old (approx.)
Blood				
acid base				
P_{CO_2}	kPa	mmHg	0.133	7.5
P_{O_2}	kPa	mmHg	0.133	7.5
Standard bicarbonate	mmol/litre	mEq/litre	Numerically	equivalent
Base excess	mmol/litre	mEq/litre	Numerically	equivalent
Glucose	mmol/litre	mg/100 ml	0.0555	18
Plasma				
Sodium	mmol/litre	mEq/litre	Numerically equivalent	
Potassium	mmol/litre	mEq/litre	Numerically equivalent	
Magnesium	mmol/litre	mEq/litre	0.5	2
Chloride	mmol/litre	mEq/litre	Numerically equivalent	
Phosphate (inorganic)	mmol/litre	mEq/litre	0.323	3.0
Creatinine	μmol/litre	mg/100 ml	88.4	0.01
Urea	mmol/litre	mg/100 ml	0.166	6.0
Serum				
Calcium	mmol/litre	mg/100 ml	0.25	4.0
Iron	μmol/litre	μg/100 ml	0.179	5.6
Bilirubin	μmol/litre	mg/100 ml	17.1	0.06
Cholesterol	mmol/litre	mg/100 ml	0.0259	39
Total proteins	g/litre	g/100 ml	10.0	0.1
Albumin	g/litre	g/100 ml	10.0	0.1
Globulin	g/litre	g/100 ml	10.0	0.1

Recommended reading

The reader may wish to study certain aspects of anaesthesia in more detail. In this event, the following list of reference books, although by no means exhaustive, may prove helpful.

Atkinson, R. S., Rushman, G. B. & Lee, J. A. (1977) *A Synopsis of Anaesthesia*. 8th edn. Bristol: Wright.

Bromage, P. R. (1954) *Spinal Epidural Analgesia*. Edinburgh: Livingstone.

Campbell, E. J. M., Sykes, M. K. & McNicol, M. W. (1977) *Respiratory Failure*. 2nd edn. London: Blackwell.

Davenport, H. T. (1978) *Paediatric Anaesthesia*. 2nd edn. London: Heinemann.

Gray, T. C. & Nunn, J. F. (1979) *General Anaesthesia*. 4th edn. London: Butterworth.

Hunter, A. R. & Bush, G. H. (1970) *General Anaesthesia for Dental Surgery*. Altrincham: Sherratt.

Macintosh, Sir Robert & Lee, J. A. (1973) *Lumbar Puncture and Spinal Analgesia*. 3rd edn. Edinburgh: Livingstone.

Macintosh, Sir Robert & Mushin, W. W. (1954) *Local Anaesthesia: Brachial Plexus*. 3rd edn. Edinburgh: Livingstone.

Moir, D. D. (1976) *Obstetric Anaesthesia and Analgesia*. London: Baillière Tindall.

Nunn, J. F. (1977) *Applied Respiratory Physiology*. 2nd edn. London: Butterworth.

Wood-Smith, F. S., Stewart, H. C. & Vickers, M. D. (1978) *Drugs in Anaesthetic Practice*. London: Butterworth.

Index